DISCLAIMER

This book has been withdrawn from the Health Library
because it has been superseded by a more recent edition
and/or is in poor physical condition. Neither the Library
nor the University accepts responsibility for the
currency, accuracy, or reliability of the information
contained in items withdrawn from library stock.

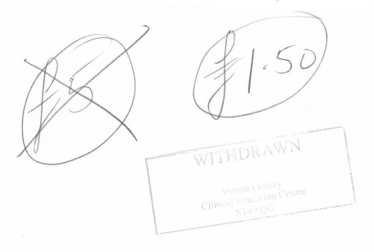

TREATMENT MANUAL FOR ANOREXIA NERVOSA

TREATMENT MANUAL FOR ANOREXIA NERVOSA
A Family-Based Approach

James Lock
Daniel le Grange
W. Stewart Agras
Christopher Dare

Foreword by Gerald Russell

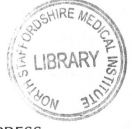

THE GUILFORD PRESS
New York   London

© 2001 The Guilford Press
A Division of Guilford Publications, Inc.
72 Spring Street, New York, NY 10012
www.guilford.com

Printed in the United States of America

This book is printed on acid-free paper.

Last digit is print number: 9 8 7 6 5 4 3 2 1

Library of Congress Cataloging-in-Publication Data

Treatment manual for anorexia nervosa : a family-based approach /
   James Lock . . . [et al.]; foreword by Gerald Russell.
     p. cm.
   Includes bibliographical references and index.
   ISBN 1-57230-607-6
    1. Anorexia nervosa—Handbooks, manuals, etc. 2. Anorexia
nervosa—Patients—Family relationships—Handbooks, manuals,
etc. 3. Family psychotherapy—Handbooks, manuals,
etc. I. Lock, James.

RC552.A5 T745 2001
616.85'262—dc21

                                      00-061757

In my view of the undoubted psychological aspects [of the disorder], it would be equally regrettable to ignore or misinterpret the patients' psychological surroundings. None should be surprised to note that I always consider the morbid state of the hysterical patient side by side with the preoccupations of her relatives.

—E. C. LASEGUE (1873)

About the Authors

James Lock, MD, PhD, is Assistant Professor of Child Psychiatry in the Department of Psychiatry and Behavioral Sciences at Stanford University School of Medicine. He is also the chief of psychiatric inpatient services at Lucile Salter Packard Children's Hospital at Stanford. Dr. Lock was trained in general psychiatry at the University of California at Los Angeles Medical Center and in child and adolescent psychiatry at the University of California at Davis. He is the author of numerous scientific and clinical papers on the subject of eating disorders in adolescents and has spent the majority of his clinical and scientific career in treating adolescents with anorexia nervosa. Dr. Lock currently holds a Career Development Award from the National Institute of Mental Health in the area of anorexia nervosa psychotherapy research.

Daniel le Grange, PhD, is Assistant Professor of Psychiatry and Director of the Eating Disorders Program in the Department of Psychiatry at the University of Chicago. He received his doctoral education at the Institute of Psychiatry, University of London, and trained in family therapy for adolescent anorexia nervosa at the Maudsley Hospital in London. At the Maudsley Hospital, he participated in some of the original family therapy studies for anorexia nervosa. Dr. le Grange is the author of numerous research and clinical articles on the subject of family treatment for adolescent anorexia nervosa. At present, he is actively involved in research into treatment and cross-cultural aspects of eating disorders.

W. Stewart Agras, MD, received his medical training at the University College, London, and his psychiatry training at McGill University in Montreal. He is Professor and Associate Chair of the Department of Psychiatry and Behavioral Sciences at Stanford University School of Medicine. For most of his career his research interests have been in the psychotherapeutic treatment of eating disorders. He is an internationally known scholar and has published several hundred scientific articles and clinical papers on eating-disorder research and treatment. He serves on numerous editorial boards and was the first president of the Society for Behavioral Medicine. Dr. Agras is also a Fellow of the Royal College of Physicians.

Christopher Dare, MD, is a Reader in Psychotherapy and the Head of the Section of Psychotherapy at the Department of Psychiatry, Institute of Psychiatry, at the Maudsley Hospital in London. He is also Consultant Psychiatrist to the Adolescent Eating Disorder Clinic, South London, and Maudsley NHS Trust. Dr. Dare was among the original authors of the first empirical studies to support family treatment for adolescents with anorexia nervosa. Subsequently, he has published numerous research and clinical articles on the role of family treatment in adolescent anorexia nervosa and is an internationally recognized expert in this field.

Acknowledgments

The authors would like to acknowledge the contributions of a number of others in the development of this treatment manual. The important and ongoing work of the clinicians and researchers at the Maudsley Hospital in London has been fundamental in the initial development and empirical testing of the treatment approach used in the manual. Among those we are most indebted to are Ivan Eisler, Gerald Russell, Elizabeth Dodge, George Szmukler, and Matthew Hodes. For specific development and piloting of the manualized treatment, we are grateful to the researchers and clinicians at the Department of Psychiatry and Behavioral Sciences at Stanford University, particularly Hans Steiner and Helena Kraemer. We would also like to thank the families who participated in the manualization process and who generously allowed us to use excerpts from their treatment. In addition, Dr. Lock's work has been supported by NIMH Career Development Award No. K08 MH01457-02.

Finally, on a personal note, we wish to thank our families for supporting our efforts on this project.

Foreword

Newcomers to anorexia nervosa may be surprised to learn that family therapy as presented in the *Treatment Manual for Anorexia Nervosa: A Family-Based Approach*, constitutes a radical break from the traditional treatment of the illness. The basic premise of this form of family therapy is that the parents should be seen as a most useful resource in the treatment of adolescents with anorexia nervosa. This view is the converse of that taken by our medical forefathers. William Gull described anorexia nervosa in 1874 and gave it its name. As a physician, he understood the need to correct the patient's malnutrition but he was scathing about her family:

> The patients should be fed at regular intervals, and surrounded by persons who would have moral control over them; relations and friends being generally the worst attendants. (p. 23)

A few years later (1882—1885), Jean-Martin Charcot, physician to the Salpêtrière in Paris, enunciated his approach to the moral (psychological) treatment of anorexia nervosa. He stressed the "curative influence of isolation," which entailed suppression of all visits from relations or friends. In particular, he believed that the presence of parents would "effectively check all treatment" (Silverman, 1997). In France, the separation (not isolation) of the patient from her parents remains a component of most inpatient treatment programs. In Britain and the United States, such a draconian approach would require quasi-legal intervention. But the culture of blaming the family for the patient's illness remains commonplace even to this day.

The beginnings of family therapy for anorexia nervosa can be traced back to the 1970s. The pioneers were Salvador Minuchin and Mara Selvini Palazzoli, but they too described abnormal interactions within the families, implying causality albeit in a noncritical manner. It remained for Christopher Dare to develop a new form of family therapy, that which is set forth in this manual. Lock and colleagues acknowledge unstintingly the fundamental work originating from the Maudsley Hospital in London, where basic research has been undertaken since the 1980s demonstrating the enduring benefits of family therapy for adolescents with anorexia nervosa. The Maudsley was also the cradle for the specific brand of family therapy devised by Dare.

This manual skillfully describes the principles that underpin Dare's form of family therapy. The parents are viewed as the best treatment resource toward achieving the patient's recovery. They are encouraged to take control of their ill daughter's food intake while the therapist acknowledges the enormous difficulties of this task. The therapist focuses on the need to restore the patient's weight to normal, at least during the initial, arduous phases of treatment. The therapy is designed to take into account the adolescent developmental process, but only later on, after the patient achieves a stable weight, does the therapist address the key developmental issues. Central to Dare's family therapy is the exoneration of the parents from blame for the illness: they are congratulated on their earlier parenting skills and encouraged to work out for themselves how best to refeed their anorexic child. An essential principle of the therapy therefore is an agnostic view of the cause of the illness, which holds the family not guilty but utilizes it as the best available means for recovery. Another key feature of the therapy is the technique of raising the parents' level of anxiety so as to engage them fully in treatment. The therapist does this by conveying the seriousness of their daughter's illness, including the risk of dying.

This manual builds on the key principles by providing rich practical advice on how best to achieve the stated aims. The patient's own compliance is usually obtained with difficulty; after all, she is required to gain weight, and this is the exact opposite of her wishes. Care is taken to avoid directing criticism at her. A valuable technique is a form of benevolent dissociation shared by the therapist, the family, and the patient. An artificial separation is established between the patient herself and her illness. She is given full support as a developing adolescent but she is told the anorexia nervosa must be attacked and defeated.

This manual contains gems of therapeutic practice, only a few of which can be mentioned. To promote early engagement, the family receives an initial telephone call from the therapist to whom the patient has been referred. There follows a confirmation letter stressing the seriousness of the illness and the need for all the family to attend to the first interview, as well as a telephone reminder the evening before the first appointment. It is pleasing to note the injunction that the parents first be interviewed separately from the child in order to maximize the information disclosed. Common difficulties are anticipated, such as the beguiling request from the parents to discover the "underlying causes" of the illness before tackling their task of refeeding. Advice is also given on how best to grapple with the complications of family structure resulting from divorce and remarriage.

The design of this manual is systematic and conforms to the three phases of therapy. Each phase consists of a sequence of goals and the text describes their rationale and ways of achieving them. The manual is designed so as to alternate a chapter of advice to the therapist with a chapter on the session in action, reporting verbatim the exchanges between family members, patient, and therapist. All the components of the family therapy are covered in such a way as to keep the therapist on track. This design brings the sessions alive and makes for compelling reading.

Treatment Manual for Anorexia Nervosa will prove to be indispensable to trainees in family therapy, and practicing therapists will also learn a great deal from it. When Christopher Dare, Ivan Eisler, and their colleagues published their method of family therapy for anorexia nervosa (Dare, Eisler, Russell, & Szmukler, 1990) they probably left some loose ends. These loose ends have been assiduously tied together in this manual, which will come to be recognized as a valuable contribution to the literature.

GERALD RUSSELL, MD

References

Dare, C., Eisler, I., Russell, G. F. M., & Szmukler, G. I. (1990). The clinical and theoretical impact of a controlled trial of family therapy in anorexia nervosa. *Journal of Marital and Family Therapy, 16,* 39–57.

Gull, W. W. (1874). Anorexia nervosa (apepsia hysterica, anorexia hysterica). *Transactions of the Clinical Society of London, 7,* 22–28.

Silverman, J. A. (1997). Charcot's comments on the therapeutic role of isolation in the treatment of anorexia nervosa. *International Journal of Eating Disorders, 21,* 295–298.

Preface

*W*e offer this book to clinicians who work with adolescents with anorexia nervosa. The manual is based on a family therapy originally developed by Christopher Dare and Ivan Eisler at the Maudsley Hospital in London. Their creative blend of family therapy approaches led to a specific and focused therapy appropriate for adolescents with anorexia nervosa. Furthermore, for over a decade, the Maudsley group has consistently demonstrated through empirical studies the effectiveness of this treatment approach with this patient population.

Until now, training in this approach has been available to a limited number of students and professionals who could travel and work with the Maudsley group in London. With the development of this manual, this treatment approach becomes more accessible to other clinicians working with adolescents with anorexia nervosa.

All of the authors have spent a major portion of their careers in clinical and research efforts devoted to helping patients and families to cope with this devastating illness, and as such, are aware of the complexities and ambiguities with which this illness presents. Though these may have seemed to be overwhelming challenges to developing a manualized approach, anorexia nervosa is just the type of illness where the guidance that a treatment manual provides is essential so the clinician can stay on a steady course. This book provides an overall structure for treatment that specifies goals, identifies strategies for specific problems, presents a time course, and provides the clinicians with tools to assess progress and outcomes. The therapeutic approach is not rigid, but provides clinicians with the necessary tools to be successful in the context of their own particular treatment styles and settings. In addition, success with this treatment, as with any other, depends on the basic psychotherapeutic skills of empathy, rapport, and communication of understanding and support of the patient and family. Our main hope in developing this manual is that by making this approach available in a manualized format, more adolescents with anorexia nervosa will recover sooner from their illness so they can resume the normal trajectory of their lives.

Contents

1

Introduction and Background Information on Anorexia Nervosa

Purpose of This Manual

This manual contains background information essential to the understanding of adolescent anorexia nervosa (AN) and its treatment with a family-based approach. It presents a treatment program, including the details of specific sessions and phases of therapy, that is based on research that has demonstrated effectiveness. The manual derives from several controlled trials of family treatment for AN, initially done at the Maudsley Hospital, London, and subsequently studied at Stanford University's Department of Psychiatry, Child Division, and at Lucile Salter Packard Children's Hospital (Eisler et al., 1997; Le Grange, 1993; Le Grange, Eisler, Dare, & Russell, 1992; Russell, Szmukler, Dare, & Eisler, 1987). This manual is intended for use by qualified therapists who have experience in the assessment and treatment of eating disorders in adolescents. It may also be used by therapists in training under the guidance of experienced clinicians. It is not intended as a self-help manual. The treatment described should be conducted with appropriate consultation and involvement of professionals in pediatric medicine, nutrition, and child psychiatry. This manual is explicitly not to be used for research purposes without further consultation with the au-

1

thors. Clinical response to these interventions is not guaranteed nor implied by the use of this manual.

The overall perspective of this therapeutic approach is to see the family as a resource in the treatment of adolescent patients with AN. Mobilizing parents and family members as a resource is the most important theoretical position that sets this approach apart from other family and individual therapies for AN. Parents play an important role throughout the three phases of this treatment. Thus, the first phase of treatment attempts to reinvigorate parental roles in the family system, particularly as they are related to the patient's eating behaviors. This is considered the key therapeutic maneuver in this phase of family treatment. Therapy is almost entirely focused on the eating disorder and its symptoms and begins with a family meal. The therapist's goal in this phase is to develop a strong parental alliance on the one hand and to align the patient with a peer or sibling subsystem. The families are encouraged to work out for themselves the best way to refeed their anorexic child. The second phase begins when the patient accepts parental demands to increase food intake and begins to experience steady weight gain. At this point, family therapy focuses on other family problems and the effect these issues have on the parents' task of supporting steady weight gain in the patient. The third phase begins when the patient achieves a relatively stable weight and self-starvation has abated. The central theme is the establishment of a healthy adolescent relationship with parents in which AN does not constitute the basis of the interaction. This entails working toward increased personal autonomy for the adolescent, more appropriate family boundaries, and the need for the parents to reorganize their life together as their adolescent children become more independent.

The manual consists of 14 chapters. Chapter 1 provides an introduction and overview of AN in adolescents. Chapter 2 provides a specific introduction to family therapy for AN and provides a more detailed introduction to the therapy that is the subject of the remaining chapters. Chapters 3–13 provide detailed instructions for how to conduct a family-based therapy for AN based on the Maudsley method developed by Christopher Dare and Ivan Eisler. Particular emphasis is devoted to the initial sessions because these sessions set the tone and therapeutic style that will be employed throughout the treatment. In these chapters, we provide descriptions of what therapeutic maneuvers the therapist is to undertake and why, as well as illustrations of each of these maneuvers. In addition, we present examples illustrating the series of therapeutic maneuvers as they are integrated in a session. We also provide a complete case illustration in Chapter 14.

In this introductory chapter we focus on providing general background material on AN. We refer to the pertinent research literature, describe the way the illness presents in adolescents, and discuss treatment options and prognosis.

Overview of Anorexia Nervosa in Adolescents

AN is a serious psychiatric illness with a prevalence estimated at 0.48% among girls aged 15–19 and 9 to 10 times more common in girls than in boys (Lucas, Beard, O'Fallon, & Kurland, 1991). In AN, pathological thoughts and behaviors about food and weight, as well as emotions concerning appearance, eating, and food, co-occur. These thoughts, feelings and behaviors lead to changes in body composition and functioning that are the direct result of starvation. Treatment of AN is complex and requires attention to broad psychiatric, medical, and nutritional aspects of the disease (American Psychiatric Association, 2000; Steiner & Lock, 1998). In adolescents, the illness severely affects physical, emotional, and social development (Fisher et al., 1995; Le Grange, Eisler, Dare, & Russell, 1992; Lucas, Beard, O'Fallon, & Kurland, 1991; Yates, 1990). Unfortunately, AN becomes a chronic illness for many patients. Multiple hospitalizations and prolonged treatment are often the rule for many patients with AN (Kreipe, Churchill, & Strauss, 1989; Kreipe & Uphoff, 1992; Society for Adolescent Medicine, 1995; Steiner, Mazer, & Litt, 1990; Yager et al., 1993).

Epidemiology and Comorbidity

Lucas et al. (1991) performed a population-based incidence study of AN in Rochester, Minnesota, over a 50-year span (1935–1984). The incidence rate for females decreased from 16.6 per 100,000 person-years between 1935 and 1939 to 7 between 1950 and 1954 and increased to 26.3 between 1980 and 1984. The incidence rates for women over 20 years remained constant, but there was a significant increase for females aged 15–24. The overall age-adjusted incidence rate was 14.6 for females and 1.8 for males.

There is a fair amount of evidence that suggests that AN often co-occurs with other psychiatric disorders. Depression is a common comorbid diagnosis, with a lifetime prevalence rate of up to 63% in some studies (Herzog, Keller, Sacks, Yeh, & Lavori, 1992). In addition, Smith, Nasserbakht, Feldman, and Steiner (1993) found that with persistent AN, there was a high incidence of anxiety disorders. In particular, Rastam (1992) found that 35% of patients with AN also suffer from comorbid obsessive–compulsive disorder. A moderate degree of overlap between avoidant personality disorder and AN has been shown in adult patients (Herzog, Keller, & Lavori, 1992), but it is unclear if this will be true for adolescents or children.

Etiology and Risks for Development

The causes of AN are unknown. Most clinicians and researchers agree, however, that AN has multiple determinants (Garfinkel & Garner, 1982; Garner, 1993; Hsu, 1990; Lask & Bryant-Waugh, 1992) that emerge in a developmental sequence (Crisp, Hsu, Harding, & Hartshorn, 1980; Steiner & Lock, 1998; Steiner, Sanders, & Ryst, 1995). Onset usually occurs during adolescence, the mean age being 17 (Hsu, 1990). Most accounts of eating disorders emphasize the individual's difficulty negotiating the developmental demands of adolescence. Recent research focuses on antecedent risks for these disorders (Childress, Maloney, Schur, Sanders & Steiner, 1999; Killen, Hayward, & Litt, 1992; Steiner & Lock, 1998; Sharpe, Ryst, Hinshaw, & Steiner, 1998; Stice, Agras, & Hammer 1999). These studies recognize that premorbid histories identify probable antecedent risks for the disorders. For example, in a short-term prospective study, Attie and Brooks-Gunn (1989) tested the hypothesis that the development of eating problems represents an accommodation to puberty. They followed a group of girls from 7th through 10th grades for 2 years. They found that eating problems emerged in response to pubertal change, especially fat accumulation. Girls who felt most negatively about their bodies at puberty were at highest risk for the development of eating difficulties after initial eating-problem scores were taken into account

There also appear to be some context-dependent risk factors associated with the development of AN. Among these are teasing by peers (Fabian & Thompson, 1989), discomfort in discussing problems with parents (Larson, 1991), maternal preoccupation with restricting dietary intake (Hill, Weaver, & Blundell, 1990), and acculturation to the Western values in immigrants (Pumariega, 1986; Steinhausen, 1995). In addition, a variety of associated risks have been identified; being female and having a pear-shaped body and a body mass index high in fat are identified as constituting risk (Radke-Sharpe, Whitney-Saltiel, & Rodin, 1990). In some studies, a high incidence of sexual abuse has been reported by women diagnosed with an eating disorder (Palmer, Oppenheimer, Dignon, Cholnor, & Howells, 1990; Rorty, Yager, & Rossotto, 1994).

There is some evidence for the familial clustering of eating disorders (e.g., Strober, 1990) and eating attitudes (Rutherford, McGuffin, Kutz, & Murray, 1993). This may suggest a role for heritable causation, but there are no adequate longitudinal studies controlling shared and nonshared environments. On the other hand, studies of families with eating disorders find distinct characteristics by both self-report and observational methods (Steiger, Leung, & Houle, 1992). Families of patients with AN appear more controlled and organized, whereas families of bulimic patients are more chaotic, conflicted, and critical.

In addition to these risks, clinicians and researchers also see an important role for the patient's motivational state in the genesis of AN. Crisp's psychobiological perspective suggests that the symptoms of starvation and emaciation represent attempts to cope with the demands of adolescence by regression to an earlier developmental level (Crisp, 1997; Crisp et al., 1980). Bruch's (1973) psychodynamic formulation conceives of the patient as becoming overwhelmed by feelings of ineffectiveness and emptiness and concomitant inability to access her own thoughts, feelings, and beliefs. Experiencing the self as lacking "a core personality" (Bruch, 1995, p. 10), she experiences the demands of puberty as overwhelming and retreats to rigid preoccupation with food and eating. Although these theories have not been tested, both support the general clinical impression that AN may represent a failed attempt to manage developmental tasks of adolescence.

Efforts are also being made to reconcile biological deficits and developmental factors with a psychodynamic understanding of eating disorders. Children at risk for the development of eating disorders may be vulnerable because of appetite and satiety dysregulation (Steiner, Smith, Rosenkrantz, & Litt, 1991; Stice et al., 1999). In addition, temperamental traits are important. For example, Strober (1991) emphasizes that patients with AN commonly express traits of harm avoidance, low novelty seeking, and high reward dependence—traits heavily influenced by genetic factors (Cloninger, 1986, 1987, 1988). These traits are at odds with the developmental tasks associated with puberty that require risk taking and independence. Adolescents without these abilities may retreat from demands for which they feel ill prepared. In addition to these temperamental factors, personality differences that may serve as precipitants to an eating disorder have been noted in persons with AN. Patients with AN are typically anxious, inhibited, and overcontrolled (e.g., Shaw, Ryst, & Steiner, 1997; Casper, Hedeker, & McClough, 1992; Leon, Fulkerson, Perry, & Cudeck, 1992).

Treatment

One of the major complications of AN is the severe medical problems that commonly co-occur with the illness. The short- and long-term medical complications of AN in adolescents are well known (Fisher et al., 1995; Palla & Litt, 1988). Changes in growth hormone, hypothalamic hypogonadism, bone marrow hypoplasia, structural abnormalities of the brain, cardiac dysfunction, and gastrointestinal difficulties are all common. Recent studies continue to document that the most significant medical problems for adolescents that differ from those of adults are the potential for significant growth retardation, pubertal delay or interruption, and peak bone mass reduction. Risks of death as a result of complications of AN are estimated at 6–15% (Steinhausen, Rauss-Mason, & Seidel, 1991, 1993), with half the deaths resulting from suicide.

Usual treatment of AN requires a multidisciplinary approach. Guidelines for the psychiatric and medical treatment of AN are published (American Psychiatric Association, 2000; Society for Adolescent Medicine, 1995). Overall, results of all treatment types are modest to moderate (Kreipe & Uphoff, 1992).

Inpatient Treatments

The role of hospitalization for AN has changed dramatically over the past 10 years, at least in the United States. Currently, hospital treatment in the United States is limited to brief acute weight restoration and refeeding. However, low discharge weight appears to confer unnecessary risk for relapse and poor prognosis (Baran, Weftzer, & Kaye, 1995). Inpatient treatment studies of young adults suggest a continued role for this modality of treatment for severe cases. Studies of intensive day treatment programs also suggest that they may be an effective alternative to inpatient treatment for some patients with AN, but specific studies of children and adolescents in such settings are lacking (Howard, Evans, Quintero-Howard, Bowers, & Andersen, 1999). A variety of investigators have published reports on the effectiveness of inpatient hospitalization for acute treatment of AN. Hospital-based treatments have been studied by McKenzie (1992), who reported that about 40% of hospitalized patients with AN are readmitted at least once and that these patients spent more time in the hospital with each admission than any other patient group with nonorganic disorders. Both short-term and longer term studies suggest that inpatient treatment may be effective. For example, Bossert (1988) found overall clinical improvement in 16 female patients after an average 3-month inpatient treatment using a behavioral approach, whereas Jenkins (1987), using a strict behavioral refeeding program for a 6-month treatment period, found that 70% showed continued improvement at a 3-year follow-up. These studies demonstrate that, using a variety of clinical approaches, inpatient treatment is likely to result in clinical improvement. However, because of increasing pressure to reduce the use of inpatient treatment due to high cost and the disruption to the adolescent's usual life, outpatient alternatives are increasingly important. One of the goals of our manualized family-based treatment program is to prevent or reduce the need for inpatient treatment by assisting the family in the outpatient setting to refeed their child. If these efforts fail, hospitalization is still an important treatment option.

Outpatient Psychosocial Treatments

Outpatient treatment approaches for AN are also being explored, including individual, family, and group therapy. A number of preliminary controlled and uncontrolled treatment trials of anorexia nervosa took place in the 1970s and 1980s. Minuchin, Baker, Rosman, Milman, and Todd (1978) reported a good outcome in 80% of cases using structural family therapy. In addition, Stierlin and Weber (1989) published results of a study using family treatment with a group of 42 families without a controlled group. At follow-up they found that about two-thirds were improved. These results came from treatments that were quite brief—most lasting about 6 months. Only 25% of cases received treatment that lasted more than 1 year. The average was only six sessions of treatment per family (Stierlin & Weber, 1989). Thus these early uncontrolled studies suggested that effective treatment of AN using a family approach could be accomplished in a relatively short time in low-intensity treatment.

There are few comparisons between inpatient and outpatient treatment approaches to AN. In a study of 85 adult female patients admitted to a hospital for AN, Kennedy et al. (1989) found that they did not differ significantly in terms of overall psychopathology, weight gain, and attitudes from outpatients with AN. This suggests that outpatient care may be as effective as inpatient care (Kennedy et al., 1989). This question was addressed by Gowers, Norton, Halek, and Crisp (1994), who compared 90 adult patients with AN randomized into four treatment groups (one inpatient, two outpatient, and one assessment-only) and found that at the end of treatment there were no differences in the treatment groups in terms of weight or body mass index, except that the assessment-only group fared worse (Gowers et al., 1994). Although these studies were of adult patients with AN, they suggest that alternatives to hospitalization might be possible in treating adolescents with AN.

In more recent years, there have been nine published trials of outpatient psychotherapy for AN (see Table 1.1); about 300 patients or patients and their families were treated in these controlled trials. The earliest of these trials was in 1987, and the most recent trial is in press. Treatment approaches included nutritional advice, family therapy of different types, individual therapy, group therapy, and cognitive and behavioral approaches. The summary of outcomes reported in Table

1.1 are characterized using the best information available to allow stratification into modified Morgan–Russell outcome categories of physical measures of recovery: good (return to normal weight and menses), intermediate (return to normal weight or menses), or poor (below normal weight and no return of menses). Percentages reported are the proportion of patients who recovered to a level of good or intermediate using these criteria. The range is from 39% to 63%. Most scores fall into the 60% range, a moderately high proportion of cases overall. However, there appears to be little relationship between outcome and either treatment duration or treatment intensity as we defined them. For example, Robin and colleagues (Robin, Siegel, Moye, & Tice, 1994; Robin et al., 1999) whose program was of both long duration and high intensity, achieved very little difference in outcomes compared with those of Crisp et al. (1991) or Le Grange, Eisler, Dare, and Russell (1992), programs which were of much shorter duration and of lower intensity. These studies suggest that for AN in general, a variety of outpatient treatment approaches can be somewhat effective, including cognitive-behavioral, behavioral, and family therapy. Definitive conclusions about treatment effectiveness are limited in many of the studies cited because of low study power secondary to small sample sizes.

At the same time, it should be noted that the majority of studies used family therapy as the studied treatment, especially for AN in younger patients. Specific research in adolescent AN has found the most promising results in the treatment effectiveness of family therapy. (We review these studies in more detail in Chapter 2.) Russell et al. (1987) compared family therapy of the type described in this manual with a form of individual therapy that emphasized support, education, and problem solving. Outcomes at 1-year follow-up were decidedly superior for the younger patients who received family therapy and for the older patients who received individual therapy (Russell et al., 1987). Follow-up data suggests that these outcomes continue to hold up at 5 years after treatment (Eisler et al., 1997). Others report similar findings using somewhat different methodologies (Robin et al., 1994, 1999).

Another interesting aspect of the controlled trials is the question of how much treatment should be given and how long treatment should last for AN. The findings of the available trials are particularly pertinent for the design of this treatment manual because a decision about both the duration and the frequency of treatment had to be made. Table 1.1 includes a summary of treatment duration and intensity for all published studies. First, approaching the question of duration of treatment, the length of treatment intervention ranged from 5

TABLE 1.1. Randomized Psychotherapy Treatment Trials in Anorexia Nervosa

Study	Type of therapy	Number of subjects	Duration of therapy	Intensity of therapy (number of sessions)	Percent with moderate and good results at 1-year outcomes (Morgan–Russell)
Hall & Crisp (1987)	Dietary advice or combined family and individual therapy	30	6–12 months	12	40%[a]
Russell et al. (1987)	Family therapy and individual therapy	57	6–12 months	Family: 10.5 ($SD = 8.9$) Individual: 15.9 ($SD = 8.5$)	39%
Channon et al. (1989)	Cognitive-behavioral treatment, standard behavioral treatment, and no treatment	24	6–12 months	24	[b]
Crisp et al. (1991)	Inpatient with outpatient follow-up, outpatient only (individual, family, nutrition), or outpatient group assessment	90	10 months	Outpatient: 12 Group: 10	60%
Le Grange, Eisler, Dare, & Russell (1992)	Whole family and separated family therapy	18	6 months	Whole family: 8.9 ($SD = 4.12$) Separated family 9.3 ($SD = 4.1$)	68%
Robin et al. (1994, 1999)	Family therapy or individual and family support	37	12–18 months	36–54	68%
Treasure et al. (1995)	Cognitive-analytic therapy and educational therapy	30	5 months	20	63%
Eisler et al. (in press)	Conjoint family therapy vs. separated family therapy	40	12 months	18.9 ($SD = 6.5$)	63%

[a]Based on percentage who had return of menses only.
[b]Could not be calculated based on available information. Overall improvement in treatment groups was reported as significant.

9

months (Treasure et al., 1995) to 18 months (Robin et al., 1994, 1999). Most treatments lasted between 6 months and 12 months. According to the published results, all effective treatments appeared to have similar effects, at least on weight and menstrual status, regardless of duration of treatment.

Duration of treatment only partially accounts for outcome. It is also clear that the intensity of treatment varied in these controlled trials. The average intensity varied from weekly sessions (Treasure et al., 1995) to monthly sessions (Crisp et al., 1991; Hall & Crisp, 1987). No studies reported sessions at a frequency greater than once per week, even when different types of therapies were combined (e.g., Robin et al., 1994, 1999). When these sessions are averaged over a year, one finds that a mean of about 18 sessions per year were provided in these controlled studies. This approximates the number of sessions (20 sessions) that we describe in the manual for a treatment duration of 1 year.

Medication Treatments

There are a few studies of medication treatment for AN, most of which examine adult samples (Garfinkel & Garner, 1987). During periods of acute medical compromise, psychopharmacological agents are of limited use. Medications most frequently used include antidepressants and low-dose neuroleptics. Low-dose neuroleptics are purportedly used to address severe obsessional thinking, anxiety, and psychotic-like thinking. However, there is little evidence that they help with those symptoms or behaviors associated with body shape and weight. Many older small studies have demonstrated few significant improvements in patients as a result of psychopharmacological intervention (Agras & Kraemer, 1983). More recent studies have explored the role of serotonin reuptake inhibitors in the treatment of AN in terms of relapse prevention, but systematic studies are not yet available (Gwirtzman, Guze, & Yager, 1990). The role of psychopharmacological treatment of comorbid disorders such as depression and anxiety, on the other hand, seems to be indicated. The treatment proposed in this manual allows for the use of these agents for comorbid conditions.

Outcomes for Patients with Anorexia Nervosa

A variety of studies have looked at the short, intermediate, and long-term outcomes of patients with AN after treatment. Most of these studies are of adult populations, although many of the patients in these studies presumably had AN as teenagers. Studies have generally demonstrated that approximately half have good outcomes, one-fourth have intermediate outcomes, and about one-fourth do poorly (Herzog et al., 1999; Ratnasuriya, Eisler, & Szmukler, 1991; Smith et al., 1993; Steinhausen et al., 1991, 1993; vand der-ham, Van Strien, & van England, 1994; Walford & McCune, 1991). Less than 5% of the patients died (Yager et al., 1993), but death rates as high as 20% have been reported in chronically ill adults with AN (Ratnasuriya et al., 1991). Assessment of recovery in these studies has been generally confined to measures of weight and nutritional rehabilitation, but some studies indicate that other psychiatric and social aspects of the illness persist. Herzog et al. (1996) reported that the bulimic subtype of anorectic patients had a higher short-term recovery rate than restricting anorectics. Treatment compliance and personality variables may be important mediators of improved treatment outcome (Steiner et al., 1990). Higher levels of general psychopathology increase the risk of poorer treatment outcomes, though depression itself was of no predictive value in adolescent samples (Herpertz-Dalmann, Wewetzer, Schulz, & Kemschmidt, 1996).

Summary

In this chapter we reviewed the etiology, clinical presentation, treatment, and prognosis of AN, to provide general background information for the reader. We also stressed several important aspects of AN and its treatment that bear specifically on the approach used in this manual. The first of these is that AN is a disorder that primarily begins in adolescence and seems to bear some relation to difficulties associated with adolescent development. As such, approaches that take into account the developmental issues associated with adolescence are most likely to succeed. Recovery appears to be best for patients who are treated early in their course, supporting the idea that adolescent interventions should be paramount in preventing the development of a more chronic and unremitting form of the illness. In addition, although treatment approaches have not been particularly well studied, we noted that for adolescents family-based approaches appear to be superior to individual approaches. This may seem counterintuitive to some clinicians who emphasize the adolescent's need for autonomy and self-control, which is indeed an expected part of adolescent development. Instead, our approach emphasizes that the adolescent with AN is regressed and out of control and needs the help of parents to "get back on track" so that the usual work of adolescent individuation can be taken up again without the symptoms of AN. Thus families appear to be an important resource for adolescents in recovering from AN. The manualized therapy described in the following chapters takes these observations into account. That is, it is designed to specifically address the need for refeeding by parents of adolescents whose eating behavior is out of their control; it also aims to support the developing adolescent in the context of the family.

In sum, we suggest that the manualized treatment described in the following pages represents a treatment that is empirically supported, provides for a rapid and relatively short treatment schedule, and fits well within the frame of accepted treatments for AN. This treatment differs from many others in several important ways as well. Among these are: the use of the parents to help in refeeding the adolescent, the focus on refeeding until weight is recovered, and the deferring of general adolescent and family issues until the eating-disordered behavior is well under control. A more thorough discussion of the advantages of this approach is undertaken in Chapter 2.

2

Family Treatment
for Anorexia Nervosa

Specific Review of Family Therapy Literature
with Focus on Maudsley Work

AN has been in the domain of family therapists for many years now
(Dare & Eisler, 1997; Minuchin et al., 1975; Selvini Palazzoli, 1974;
Wynne, 1980). In addition, family problems have long been identified
as part of the presentation of eating disorders (Bliss & Branch, 1960;
Bruch, 1973; Gull, 1874; Morgan & Russell, 1975). In fact, according to
Dare and Eisler (1997), AN can been seen as paradigmatic for family
therapy, much as hysteria was seen for psychoanalysis and phobias for
behavior therapy. Minuchin and colleagues at the Philadelphia Child
Guidance Clinic (1975) and Salvini Palazzoli at the Milan Center (1974)
both observed specific characteristics of these families. Both emphasized the overly close nature of family relationships, the blurring of
intergenerational boundaries, and tendencies to avoid overt conflict.

Only a brief review of the range of approaches to family therapy
for AN can be presented here. We provide this review to help place the
manualized version of the Maudsley method in context. We also hope
to show how this approach incorporates elements of other approaches
in a new synthesis specifically designed to treat adolescents with AN.
Readers interested in a more thorough discussion of these other approaches are encouraged to consult the references cited in this discussion.

In the traditional model of family therapy, the patient is seen as having developed a problem in response to various external factors (e.g., genetic, physiological, familial, sociocultural, etc.). In this model, treatment is conceptualized as aimed at the individual and designed to counteract the effects of these external causative factors. Within this model, family intervention attempts to modify the problems within the family or, if necessary, to remove the child from the family (Harper, 1983). Family therapy approaches in general conceptualize the problem or symptom as belonging to the entire family. The approach is aimed at the entire family system.

Structural family therapy developed an approach to anorexia nervosa from the perspective of treating psychosomatic families (Liebman, Minuchin, & Baker, 1974; Minuchin et al., 1975). This approach sees children in such a family as being physiologically vulnerable in the context of a family, whose transactional characteristics include enmeshment, overprotectiveness, rigidity, and lack of conflict resolution. In addition, the affected child has a critical role in the family's avoidance of conflict that acts as a powerful reinforcement for symptoms. Structural interventions are designed to alter the family organization by challenging alliances between parents and children that disrupt parental effectiveness, by encouraging the development of stronger sibling subsystems, and by encouraging more open communication both within the family and with the larger social world. Using this approach with families with eating problems, Minuchin added a participant observation of a family meal in which parents are encouraged to take control of the meal. In so doing, the result is that the daughter's emotional involvement with her parents is reduced, while at the same time the parents through their work together reinforce the effectiveness of their own parental dyad. Some elements of this approach underlie the family meal used in the treatment of adolescent AN in the Maudsley model (Dare, 1985; Dare, Eisler, Russell, & Szmukler, 1990) that is manualized in this book.

Strategic family therapy has also contributed to some of the approaches that are employed in the Maudsley model. In particular, the "agnostic" view regarding etiology about the causes of psychological disorders is an important shared starting point. Haley (1973) and Madanes (1981) express this view as a lack of interest in the causes of illness; thus the scope of their proposed interventions is more circumscribed and aims at limiting the impact of symptoms on the patient and family. Strategic approaches used in this manualized family treatment for AN include prescribing behaviors with paradoxical intentions (e.g., asking a child to resist parental efforts to get her to eat in order to prevent premature compliance to parental authority) or suggesting that the patient undertake behaviors that challenge the symptom (e.g., recommending a patient eat in order to have the strength to fight her parents). Again, the Maudsley method incorporates some paradoxical injunctions in order to support the parental efforts at refeeding while also acknowledging the adolescent's need to resist these efforts.

Milan systems therapy shares characteristics with strategic and structural approaches; however, the most significant departure is in the formulation of the family as a rigidly organized homeostatic mechanism resistant to change from the outside (e.g., Selvini Palazzoli, 1974). The therapist remains neutral in this model in order to avoid provoking powerful homeostatic mechanisms that maintain the family system. Instead of making direct interventions, the therapist interviews the family, encouraging the family to become observers and challengers of their own process. End-of-session reviews are used to reframe observed patterns in ways that connote a positive view of family process. Both these techniques are adopted by Dare and Eisler (1997) in their work, as well as in this manualized format of the treatment. Specifically, as will be seen, the family is encouraged to find solutions that work for them rather than to rely on the outside authority of the therapist. In addition, the therapist makes a consistent effort to hold the family and its efforts in a positive, noncritical regard throughout the therapy.

Feminist theory has added a critical perspective on some of the structural and strategic approaches to family therapy that emphasize the therapist's hierarchical relationship to the patient and family. Feminist therapists emphasize instead the need for partnership and shared control of the therapeutic process (e.g., Madanes, 1997). Although the approach used in this manual, consistent with Dare and Eisler's work (1997), insists on the need for parental control of the anorectic child's eating early on in treatment, it also explicitly calls for developing a partnership with the healthy part of the adolescent's growth process, even if it defies parental will. The therapist aims to form a sincere partnership with both the parents in their tasks, as well as with the adolescent in hers.

Each of these schools of thought on family therapy makes contributions to the particular type and style of interventions used. Detail is provided in the "Why" sections in each chapter that illustrate the theoretical connection between the intervention and various schools of family therapy. At the same time, though, only the Maudsley model has been the subject of controlled trials (see the following section; see also, e.g., Eisler et al., 1997; Le Grange, Eisler, Dare, & Russell, 1992; Russell et al., 1987). Finally, it must be said that the theoretical mechanisms proposed for any of these therapies, including that of the Maudsley model itself, are unproven. Still, other unconfirmed theories, including Fairburn's cognitive-behavioral model of AN (Fairburn, Shafran, & Cooper, 1999), that are aimed at issues of control in adolescents with AN may account for progress in treatment while using the Maudsley model.

The Maudsley Method and the Evolution of This Manual

The research literature in Table 1.1 documents the lack of clear benefit of one type of treatment over another in AN, except for family therapy for adolescent patients, that is, patients 18 years and younger with a duration of illness of less than 3 years (Eisler et al., 1997; Le Grange, 1993; Le Grange et al., 1992; Russell et al., 1987). The Maudsley group has conducted several controlled family therapy studies since the mid-1980s. The most prominent of these is that of Russell et al. (1987), which compares treatment outcomes in outpatient AN. They have shown that, compared with older patients, younger patients improved with family therapy more than with individual therapy. A 5-year follow-up of the original cohort confirmed the maintenance of the positive outcome for the young patients who received family therapy (Eisler et al., 1997). In a controlled pilot study, the Maudsley group set out to explore the beneficial components of this family therapy, as well as to demonstrate the viability of family treatment as an outpatient therapy (Le Grange et al., 1992). In a follow-up study, they confirmed that family therapy is a viable alternative to inpatient treatment and that there is a relationship between family organization and treatment compliance and outcome (Eisler et al., 1997).

Family therapy has also been shown to be effective in controlled studies conducted by Arthur Robin and his group in Detroit. They compared a family therapy that was very similar to the Maudsley method with individual therapy in 37 adolescents who had AN and found that after 16 months, family therapy resulted in greater changes in body mass index, whereas both treatments demonstrated similar results in other measures (eating attitudes, body-shape concerns, and eating-related family conflicts; Robin et al., 1994, 1999). A 1-year follow-up of this cohort again demonstrated the superiority of family therapy in terms of greater weight gain and higher rates of resumption of menses when compared with individual therapy. Although individual therapy also proved effective, family therapy produced a faster return to health (Robin et al., 1999).

Why Use a Manual?

It is clear from this handful of controlled studies that family therapy based on the Maudsley method appears to be particularly helpful in the treatment of adolescents with AN. This manual reproduces the Maudsley approach that has proven efficacy for this specific subgroup of AN patients. There are benefits to both the therapist and the client when using a manual-based therapy. First, the structure, although flexible, ensures that the treatment procedures are sequenced in an optimal fashion and that all the components of therapy are adequately covered. Second, a manual keeps both the therapist and the client on track. Without the benefit of a manual, it is easy for a considerable amount of therapy time to be devoted to issues that are not central to the treatment of AN in adolescents. In this sense, this manual illustrates a highly focused treatment aimed at weight restoration and return to physical health. Third, the procedures described in this manual have been tested in controlled outcome studies; hence both the client and the therapist can have confidence that the treatment works.

Introduction to This Treatment Approach

The theoretical understanding or overall philosophy of the Maudsley method is that the adolescent is imbedded in the family and that the parents' involvement in therapy is vitally important for ultimate success in treatment. In AN the adolescent is seen as regressed. Therefore, parents should be involved in their offspring's treatment while showing respect and regard for the adolescent's point of view and experience. This treatment pays close attention to adolescent development and aims to guide the parents eventually to assist their adolescent with developmental tasks. In doing so, the family must defer working on other family conflicts or disagreements until the eating-disordered behaviors are resolved. Normal adolescent development is seen as having been arrested by the presence of the eating disorder. The parents are temporarily put in charge to help reduce the hold this disorder has over the adolescent's life. Once successful in this task, the parents will return control to the adolescent and assist her in the usual negotiation of predictable adolescent developmental tasks, as appropriate.

The Maudsley method differs from other treatments for adolescents in several key ways. First, as pointed out previously, the adolescent is not viewed as being in control of her behavior; instead, the eating disorder controls the adolescent. Thus in this way only the adolescent is seen as not functioning on an adolescent level but instead as a much younger child who is in need of a great deal of help from her parents. Second, the treatment aims to correct this position by improving parental control over the adolescent's eating. This control is often lost because parents might feel that they are to blame for the eating disorder or because the symptoms frighten them to the extent that they are too afraid to act decisively. Third, the Maudsley method strongly advocates that the therapist should primarily focus her or his attention on the task of weight restoration, particularly in the early parts of treatment. The Maudsley approach, as opposed to Minuchin's approach, tends to "stay with the eating disorder" for a longer time—that is, the therapist remains careful not to become distracted from the central therapeutic task, which is to keep the parents focused on refeeding their adolescent so as to free her from the control of the eating disorder.

This family therapy for adolescent AN usually proceeds through three clearly defined phases. Phase I usually lasts between 3 and 5 months, with sessions typically scheduled at weekly intervals. The spacing of sessions should be based on the patient's clinical progress. Toward Phase II, the therapist may schedule sessions every 2nd to 3rd week, whereas monthly sessions are advisable toward conclusion of treatment (Phase III). All sessions are 50 to 60 minutes in duration except for the family meal, for which the clinician should allow up to 90 minutes. In this manual, we first describe the broad goals of each phase, followed by the specific steps that should be followed in order to achieve these goals.

Phase I: Refeeding the Patient

In Phase I, the therapy is almost entirely focused on the eating disorder and includes a family meal, as described by Minuchin's group in Philadelphia (Liebman, Sargent, & Silver, 1983; Rosman, Minuchin, & Liebman, 1975). This procedure provides the therapist with an opportunity for direct observation of the familial interaction patterns while eating. With younger patients the therapist makes careful and persistent requests for united parental action directed toward eating, which is the primary concern at this point of the treatment. This permits the therapist to disclaim the notion that the parents have caused the eating problem and instead to express sympathy for the parents' plight. In addition, the therapist directs the discussion in such a way as to create and reinforce a strong alliance between parents in their efforts at refeeding their offspring on the one hand and to align the patient with the sibling subsystem on the other. This phase is particularly characterized by attempting to absolve the parents from the responsibility of causing the illness and by complimenting them as much as possible on the positive aspects of their parenting of their children. The attitude of the therapist should reflect something like the following sentiment: "You have been successful with bringing up your children to this point and in your personal and professional lives. We hope to encourage the application of the skills acquired in these earlier successes in helping you resolve the current eating problem with your daughter." The families are encouraged to work out for themselves how best to refeed their anorexic child (Eisler et al., 1997; Le Grange, 1993), while the therapist provides consistent support for these efforts at all times.

Phase II: Negotiations for a New Pattern of Relationships

The patient's surrender to the demands of her parents to increase her food intake (when steady weight gain is evident), as well as a change in the mood of the family (i.e., relief after having taken charge of the eating disorder), signal the start of Phase II of treatment. The therapist advises the parents to accept that the main task here is the return of their child to physical health. Although symptoms remain central in the discussions, weight gain with minimum tension is encouraged. In addition, all other issues that the family has had to postpone can now be brought forward for review. This review, however, occurs only in relationship to the effect these issues have on the parents in their task of assuring steady weight gain.

Phase III: Adolescent Issues and Termination

Phase III is initiated when the patient achieves a stable weight and the self-starvation has abated. The central theme here is the establishment of a healthy adolescent or young adult relationship with the parents in which the distorted eating does not constitute the basis of interaction. This entails, among other things, working toward increased personal autonomy for the adolescent and establishing more appropriate family boundaries, as well as the need for the parents to reorganize their life together after their children's prospective departure (Eisler et al., 1997; Le Grange, 1993; Le Grange et al., 1992; Russell et al., 1987).

Appropriate Candidates for This Therapy

The patients for whom this type of therapy is most appropriate are patients younger than 18 years of age with AN. For the most part, these will be adolescents who are living at home with their families. This is true in part because the therapy assumes that the family eats together and has routine access to one another by living in the same household. Because the therapy asks that parental figures assume leadership in refeeding the starving child, it is necessary that meals be routinely eaten together.

What constitutes a family is quite variable. For practical purposes, we define the family as those persons who live in the same household as the identified patient. This may mean that a family session should include nonbiologically related household members, or grandparents if they live in the home, whereas it may exclude parental figures who are not involved in the day-to-day care of the child with AN.

The therapy described in this manual therefore involves the entire family. This requires a substantial commitment on the part of parents and siblings to attend therapy sessions. It may require that siblings miss school or other activities to assure their attendance. The therapy also requires great dedication on the part of parental figures to do what is necessary to help their starving child. This may include taking time away from work, setting aside other pressing issues, and forgoing expected activities for a period. Families for whom this therapy is appropriate must be prepared to make these sacrifices.

Possible Modifications

The general perspective of this manual applies to intact families. However, this treatment manual can be modified for nonintact families depending on their status, such as reconstituted or single-parent families, or on the specifics of custodial arrangements. For instance, single parents may have to take on the task of refeeding their offspring by themselves, or they may wish to coopt the assistance of a friend or other relative. Some of these possibilities are discussed in more detail later on.

Noncompliant Families

Patients and families are not perfectly compliant with recommended treatments. This is true for all medical problems but may be especially so in families with a child who has AN. Many factors lead families to believe that there is no problem or that they cannot do anything about the problem even if they acknowledge it. Therefore, we do not expect perfect compliance with the treatments in this manual. However, the degree of noncompliance is very important. It is, after all, not possible to do family therapy unless the family is present. If the family does not on the whole make scheduled appointments, there is reason to strongly consider that this approach is not likely to be helpful. Families need to be handled supportively in any event, and the possible loss of an important resource for the patient (in this case the family) should be carefully evaluated. Do not give up too soon, as the family is the best resource that a patient has for recovery.

Weight-Recovered Patients

The therapy is designed for patients who need help with refeeding. If this is not a problem, even though the patient may still have severely distorted thinking associated with AN, it would be difficult to apply the strategies of the refeeding process discussed in Phase I of the manual. Nonetheless, it is no doubt also true that patients who are weight recovered may still require parental management of their eating patterns in order to keep from losing weight again. Patients who are partially weight recovered may still not be menstruating and therefore still require additional weight gain or persistent weight maintenance or both in order to continue to recover. These patients as a whole are appropriate candidates for treatment using this manual, but the focus will quickly move into Phase II and III interventions. This situation requires that the therapist conduct at least the first two sessions of Phase I, but these may soon be followed by sessions that address the need to continue with weight gain or to eat normally and the need for parents to supervise returning responsibility for eating back to the adolescent.

Hospitalized Patients

The question sometimes arises about the application of this type of therapy to an inpatient setting. The therapy as a whole is difficult to apply to most inpatient settings. This is true simply because the ability of the parents to take responsibility and action related to their child's refeeding process is curtailed by the fact that they cannot do this when staff and physicians are making these decisions. It is our impression, however, that the crisis of a hospitalization can be used by the therapist to increase the productive concern of parents. This concern, when productively channeled using techniques described in Session 1, can better prepare the parents to take action and responsibility when their daughter is once again returned to their care. Thus it may be appropriate for a therapist to conduct Session 1 in an inpatient setting, or to repeat the strategies employed in Session 1 with a family if a patient is rehospitalized, in order to get the family rapidly engaged in the treatment process. Crisp et al. (1991) and others have noted that the crisis of hospitalization itself does indeed motivate some families to action. We believe that this can be capitalized on at times when combined with the interventions described in Session 1.

Who Might Not Be Appropriate Candidates for This Therapy?

Bulimic Patients

It is unclear if this treatment is appropriate for adolescents with bulimia nervosa. Only one preliminary report (Dodge et al., 1995) suggests that family therapy for this clinical population may be helpful. The results of this study, however, are inconclusive. At this juncture, the manual does not provide strategies for patients who present with primary bulimia nervosa; however, we do provide some strategies for and examples of how to approach an adolescent patient with AN, binge-eating/purging type.

Other Malnourished Patients

There are reasons other than having AN for a child becoming malnourished. Some of these may indeed be behavioral in origin, such as conversion disorders, food phobias, psychotic delusions, and obsessive-compulsive disorders. There is no evidence to date that the strategies suggested in this manual are applicable to these and other types of problems with food and weight. It is our impression that, although this therapy employs many ideas from a variety of schools of thought in family therapy, it is a synthesis that may be uniquely effective for AN in adolescents.

Older Patients

One of the hallmarks of AN is the difficulty the patient has leaving home. Thus many adults with AN still live with their parents. This circumstance would seem to make this therapy also appropriate for this older population. However, Russell et al. (1987) found that older patients did better with individual therapy compared with family therapy. A follow-up study from this same group confirms this earlier trend (Eisler et al., 1997). In addition, the therapy technique presented in this manual is designed to take into account quite specifically the adolescent developmental processes. Parents still have very real control, both legal and financial, over their adolescent children in fundamentally different ways than they do with adult children, no matter how developmentally delayed or immature the adult patient may be. We recommend that this therapy be used with adolescents and, as several studies suggest (e.g., Le Grange et al., 1992; Russell et al., 1987), it will likely have the greatest impact on younger adolescents with short duration of illness.

Boys with AN are comparatively rare. Studies of adolescent family-based therapy for AN include few males. Thus, our understanding of how to best help boys with AN is quite limited. In applying the manual's treatments to boys, several suggestions may be clinically helpful. First, boys know that this illness is associated with girls and women. Some adolescent boys may feel this is an injury to their developing sense of masculinity. Therefore it is helpful if the therapist makes his/her comments as gender neutral as possible when referring to the history and prognosis of the illness. Further, it is important to try to help the family and patient value recovery from AN. This may prove to be more difficult with boys than girls because the clear physiological impact of self-starvation—amenorrhea—is not present for boys. It is useful to emphasize the possibility of growth retardation, decreased energy, and poorer academic and athletic performance in addition to the emotional sequelae of AN with these families. In this way, boys and their parents are more likely to appreciate the need for immediate refeeding.

Who Is Qualified to Use This Manual?

This manual is intended for use by qualified therapists who have experience in the assessment and treatment of eating disorders in adolescents. Therapists in training under the guidance of experienced clinicians may also use it. It is not intended as a self-help manual. The treatment described should be conducted with appropriate consultation and involvement of professionals in pediatric medicine, nutrition, and child psychiatry.

The Treatment Team

The degree of collegial (e.g., treatment team) and technical (e.g., video recording of sessions) support that the therapist requires will depend on his or her experience with families in general and eating-disordered patients in particular. This support, of course, will also depend on the setting in which the clinician operates. Few therapists, however, should aim to work completely without any support structures, as it is a complex therapeutic task, and it is relatively easy for the therapist to become caught up in family dynamics. Unlike individual psychotherapy, the clinician has to keep track of the dynamics of the entire family, and this may be overwhelming for some therapists. Even experienced family therapists can benefit from working with an observing clinician who is familiar with the physiology, psychology, and family processes related to self-starvation.

We recommend that the therapy team members include the primary clinician or team leader (e.g., a child and adolescent psychiatrist, psychologist, or social worker) and a cotherapist, whereas a consulting team could consist of a pediatrician, nurse, and nutritionist.

If possible, members of the treatment team should all be concentrated within the same facility. "Partitioning" the treatment out to various clinicians not in direct contact with the primary clinician is cause for concern. For instance, the patient may discuss a specific aspect of treatment, such as rate of weight gain, with her pediatrician who may not be intimately familiar with the primary clinician's treatment philosophy and may inadvertently provide the patient with conflicting information that may have a negative impact on the treatment process. However, the degree to which a treatment team can be assembled in the same locale without having to partition certain examinations or measurements out to others will, of course, depend on the nature of the setting in which the primary clinician operates.

The lead therapist is not always someone who can do a physical examination or who has expert nutritional knowledge. Therefore, a secondary line of clinicians, who are not directly involved in psychological treatment, may have to act as consultants to inform the lead therapist. The lead therapist has to orchestrate a system in which he or she has immediate access to the information gathered by the consultants, for example, the pediatrician. In other words, all team members have to be "on the same page." One way in which this can be achieved is for the lead therapist to establish a simple checklist such as the following that should be completed at the end of each session and then distributed to all other team members:

- What was the patient's last weight?
- What new problems were noted?
- What are your recommendations?

The Role of the Consulting Team

These are persons not ordinarily acting in the role of therapist, such as the pediatrician or nutritionist. These members are secondary in the sense that they provide clinical data to the family therapy team members. The lead therapist should coordinate regular contact with the consulting team members. These team contacts may be in the form of weekly face-to-face team meetings, weekly teleconferencing, or weekly contact through electronic mail or faxing. It is of the utmost importance that the family therapist clearly lead the treatment philosophy while taking into consideration the available clinical data. Likewise, the team members should be familiar with the family therapist's philosophy and allow this philosophy to guide their contact with the patient.

Before the therapist's first meeting with the family, arrangements would already have been made for a physical examination of the patient. This information, along with a weight chart, will be available to the therapist prior to meeting with the family. The therapist will weigh the patient during subsequent meetings and often measure height if growth is predicted. Facilities to monitor weight, height, blood chemistry, and cardiac and endocrine status should be available, or arrangements should be set up for a routine medical examination and relevant laboratory tests. This can be accomplished in a variety of ways, mainly depending on the patient's medical status; for example, regular orthostatic checks are advisable, as well as electrolyte screening if frequent purging is suspected .

What to Do If the Therapist Does Not Have Broad-Based Team Support Available

• *Work in therapy pairs.* It would be beneficial for a therapist to co-opt a colleague to work along with him or her in providing family therapy for eating disorders. Establishing a therapy pair can be advantageous in terms of mutual therapeutic insight and support. Furthermore, family dynamics can have a seductive quality and can lead to the therapist colluding with either the parents or the illness, thereby rendering treatment less effective.

• *Establish a relationship with another clinician (e.g., a pediatrician).* To prevent any miscommunication between the lead therapist and another clinician about the treatment procedures, it is best to establish a treatment relationship with just one or two pediatricians who can become familiar with this treatment approach and to whom all patients can be referred for medical monitoring. Regular meetings are recommended, especially if the lead therapist shares several patients with other clinicians. For clinicians in the United States, this arrangement may be complicated by insurer patient–therapist purchasing agreements, which ordinarily do not allow for consolidation.

• *Arrange weekly consultation or supervision with a colleague.* If it is not possible for a colleague to join the therapist in treatment, a weekly supervision or consultation should be established with a peer who would be available to review cases and provide the therapist with needed support and insights (also see the previous suggestions). Another alternative is to videotape or audiotape sessions for review with a colleague.

• *Arrange weekly team meetings or teleconferencing.* The lead therapist should take charge in organizing scheduled team meetings or weekly telephone conferencing. In addition, the lead therapist should ensure that everyone involved in the family treatment shares all relevant patient charts.

Summary

Published reports on short- and long-term follow-up of family therapy for AN using the Maudsley approach suggest that it holds great promise for short-duration illnesses among adolescents. As a specific therapy, it has roots in the rich tradition of family therapy and incorporates much from these approaches in a synthesis designed to address the developing adolescent in the context of the debilitating and life-threatening behaviors associated with AN. A manualized strategy helps properly prepared clinicians to keep focused on the role of eating-disordered behaviors in inhibiting, complicating, and disturbing the usual developmental processes of adolescence.

In this manual we present a specific approach to AN in adolescents that we believe has both empirical and clinical support based on our review of the literature. By making this treatment available in a manual, we hope that more about its appropriate clinical use will be discovered by practitioners who embrace the methods described. We recognize that no treatment works for every patient or family under all conditions. Thus we believe instead that, other than in research studies in which strict protocols are needed, the judgment of individual clinicians need apply. This is no less true for this treatment than for any other approach. Therefore, although we have endeavored to be as precise and specific as possible in the foregoing discussion, we recognize and fully expect clinicians to modify certain aspects of treatment to fit the circumstances that they find themselves practicing within. At the same time, there are certain principles of treatment that would hold, we believe, in every instance. Among these principles are: (1) an agnostic view of the cause of the illness that holds the family not guilty from the perspective of treatment; (2) a commitment to the parents as competent agents for refeeding their starved offspring; (3) the view that the entire family is an important resource in recovery; and (4) a recognition that adolescent needs for control and autonomy in areas other than weight must be respected. We also believe that the pacing of the therapy must follow the overall guideline of the phases of treatment. That is to say, the focus of the initial period of treatment must be on refeeding and weight gain under the control of the parents; not until these issues have been resolved is it advisable to proceed to discuss more general family dynamics or adolescent issues.

We include an outline of therapeutic interventions by Phase to help therapists see the pattern of the overall therapy, as well as to track their own cases (see Table 2.1). We hope that this will help the therapist who is using the manual to "keep track" of where he or she is in the treatment process and to follow the steps as outlined.

TABLE 2.1. Outline of Therapeutic Goals and Interventions

Phase I: Refeeding the patient

Session 1

There are three main goals for Session 1:

- To engage the family in the therapy.
- To obtain a history of how the AN is effecting the family.
- To obtain preliminary information about how the family functions (i.e., coalitions, authority structure, conflicts).

In order to accomplish these main goals, the therapist undertakes the following therapeutic interventions:

1. Weighing the patient.
2. Greeting the family in a sincere but grave manner.
3. Taking a history that engages each family member in the process.
4. Separating the illness from the patient.
5. Orchestrating an intense scene concerning the seriousness of the illness and difficulty in recovering.
6. Charging the parents with the task of refeeding.
7. Closing the session.

Session 2

These are three major goals for Session 2:

- To continue the assessment of the family structure and its likely impact on the ability of the parents to successfully refeed their daughter.
- To provide an opportunity for the parents to experience success in refeeding their daughter.
- To assess the family process specifically during eating.

In order to accomplish these goals, the therapist undertakes the following interventions during this session:

1. Weighing the patient.
2. Taking a history and observing the family patterns during food preparation, food serving, and family discussions about eating, especially as it relates to the patient.
3. Helping parents convince their daughter to eat at least one mouthful more than she is prepared to, *or* helping to set parents on their way to working out how they can best go about refeeding their daughter.
4. Aligning the patient with her siblings for support.
5. Closing the session.

Sessions 3–10

There are three goals for these treatment sessions:

- To keep the family focused on the eating disorder.
- To help the parents take charge of their daughter's eating.
- To mobilize siblings to support the patient.

In order to accomplish these goals, the following interventions will be appropriate to consider during the remainder of treatment for Phase I:

1. Weighing the patient at the beginning of each session.
2. Directing, redirecting, and focusing the therapeutic discussion on food and eating behaviors and their management until food, eating, and weight behaviors and concerns are relieved.
3. Discussing, supporting, and helping the parental dyad's efforts at refeeding.
4. Discussing, supporting, and helping the family to evaluate efforts of siblings to help their affected sister.
5. Continuing to modify parental and sibling criticisms.
6. Continuing to distinguish the adolescent patient and her interests from those of AN.
7. Closing all sessions with a recounting of progress.

These interventions can be applied in Sessions 3 through 10 in any order, with their momentary applicability or appropriateness determined by the family's response to the initial interventions (Sessions 1 and 2). For the purpose of clarification, however, we outline a description of each goal separately, even though in practice they may overlap to a considerable degree. Patients may require a range of sessions for completion of Phase I, sometimes as few as two to three additional sessions to as many as 10 or more.

Phase II: Negotiations for a new pattern of relationships

The major goals of Phase II treatment are:

- To maintain parental management of eating-disorder symptoms until the patient shows evidence that she is able to eat well and gain weight independently.
- To return food and weight control to the adolescent.
- To explore the relationship between adolescent developmental issues and AN.

In order to achieve these goals, the therapist needs to undertake the following interventions:

1. Weighing the patient.
2. Continuing to support and assist the parents in management of eating-disorder symptoms until the adolescent is able to eat well on her own.
3. Assisting the parents and adolescent in negotiating the return of control of eating-disorder symptoms to the adolescent.
4. Encouraging the family to examine relationships between adolescent issues and the development of AN in their adolescent.
5. Continuing to modify parental and sibling criticism of the patient, especially in relation to the task of returning control of eating to the patient.
6. Continuing to assist siblings in supporting their ill sister.
7. Continuing to highlight the differences between the adolescent's own ideas and needs and those of AN.
8. Closing sessions with positive support.

(continued)

TABLE 2.1. (*cont.*)

Although the treatment goals are the same for all needed sessions of Phase II, the emphasis of each session changes as one moves toward the end of this phase. For example, sessions may start out very similar to those of Phase I, with weight gain being the primary goal, but the emphasis will shift toward weight maintenance as control over eating is handed back to the patient. Finally, the therapist will begin to focus more on adolescent issues as she or he makes a transfer from Phase II to Phase III.

Phase III: Adolescent issues and termination

The major goals for Phase III treatment are:

- To establish that the adolescent–parent relationship no longer requires the symptoms as an idiom of communication.
- To review adolescent issues with the family and to model problem solving of these types of issues.
- To terminate treatment.

In order to accomplish these goals, the therapist undertakes the following interventions:

1. Reviewing adolescent issues with the family and modeling problem solving of these types of issues.
2. Involving the family in "review" of issues.
3. Checking how much the parents are doing as a couple.
4. Delineating and exploring adolescent themes.
5. Planning for future issues.
6. Terminating treatment.

3

Phase I: Initial Evaluation and Setting Up Treatment

*I*n this chapter we briefly review an evaluation process for adolescents with AN. This is not a standard part of the Maudsley treatment approach to AN, but we believe it will be helpful to a clinician in determining who might be considered an appropriate candidate for treatment. Initial evaluation usually consists of an interview with the adolescent, a separate interview with the parents, a medical evaluation, and possibly the use of standardized assessment instruments. Next, we describe the process that precedes the actual face-to-face therapy sessions but that is a critical part of the Maudsley method because it emphasizes the need for immediate communication of expert concern about the dilemma the patient with AN and family are facing. This entails setting up the treatment team, as well as telephone and written communications with the family detailing the high degree of seriousness and concern and the need for action to help the adolescent to recover.

Evaluation and Assessment of Adolescents with Anorexia Nervosa

Most often, adolescents with AN come to the mental health professional's attention through a referral from a concerned pediatrician. The family is often resistant to the idea that their child has an emotional problem, because she has been "perfect" throughout her upbringing. Sometimes the family also actively tries to ignore emotions, particularly conflicts, and this resistance also fuels the avoidance of a referral to a mental health professional.

Because dieting and weight concerns are part of Western culture in general and of adolescent young women in particular, it is important to distinguish between these typical and predictable concerns and those that become severe enough to warrant intervention. The standard thresholds for diagnosing AN are those described in the *DSM-IV*. The clinician should make special note that there are really two different types of criteria. The easiest for the clinician to identify are the weight and menstrual criteria. Patients who are below 85% of ideal body weight or who fail to make expected weight gains meet the weight criteria. The *DSM* also requires that three consecutive menstrual periods be missed in females who have reached menarche. These physical health thresholds are designed to ensure that patients who are diagnosed with AN truly have significant weight loss and malnutrition. The other type of criteria that are included in the *DSM* refer to the specific psychopathology of AN. These include an intense fear of weight gain, even though the patient is underweight, and an overestimation of current body mass—usually called body-image distortion. So, in order for an adolescent to be diagnosed as having AN, she must be significantly malnourished, as well as reporting fear of weight gain, while seeing her currently emaciated body as somehow still fat. In addition to these types of characteristics, it is possible that AN may be complicated by binge-eating or purging behaviors.

The clinician should expect that most adolescents with AN will minimize their symptoms. This is in part due to their distorted perception of the facts, but it also may be a conscious effort to keep clinicians from understanding their behaviors so that they will be able to continue them. For these reasons, it is imperative that the clinician also meet with others who are likely to have important information about what has been happening. The parents should be interviewed separately from their child, because much information that parents would be reluctant to confide in front of their child can be obtained this way.

Interview with the Adolescent

In an evaluation interview with an adolescent with AN, it is important to convey support and warmth while avoiding undue familiarity. Interviews can begin in a general way, with open-ended questions about the patient's family, schoolwork, interests, and activities. Gradually, the interview should be more focused on eating behaviors and problems. The therapist should look for initial triggers for the problem;

these may be of many different types. Commonly, they include other people's comments on the adolescent's weight (either remarks about being overweight or compliments on looking thinner), onset of menses, dating, family conflicts, increased pressures to achieve at school, or increased competition with peers. In addition, the therapist should carefully inquire into the manner of weight loss. Methods include restrictions on calories, fat, and meat and protein, as well as on amount of food eaten. Often the careful historian will discover that there has been a cascade of restricting activities, starting with ridding the diet of fats and sugars, then restricting proteins and meats, and finally restricting amount of food. The therapist should also inquire about other methods of weight loss, including exercise, laxative use, purging, and diuretic use. The therapist should ask about binge eating and carefully distinguish between a true binge (eating significantly more than the average person in a finite period) and a "subjective" binge (which to a person with AN might consist of two crackers and half a cup of juice). It is also important that the therapist inquire about loss of menses. Because AN is often complicated by depression, obsessive-compulsive disorder, and anxiety disorders, the interviewer should screen for these disorders as well. Throughout the interview, the therapist should be direct in style of questioning and clear about his or her interest and concern. Additional information about clinical evaluation of adolescents with AN can be found by consulting the American Psychiatric Association's *Practice Guideline for the Treatment of Eating Disorders* (APA, 2000).

Interview with the Parents

It is best to have both parents present for the parent evaluation interview, especially when both adults are involved in the care of the adolescent. Not only does this step begin to involve both parents early on with their daughter's health, but it also provides important information about both the patient and the family that otherwise might be unavailable. Sometimes one of the parents is more involved with the patient and may not see things as clearly as a more distant parent. On the other hand, if one of the parents has been overly distant, the interview can serve as a way of "pulling them in" to help with the problem. Parents should also be asked about how they see the development of AN as occurring. When did they first perceive a problem? What have they tried to do to help? Do they see other kinds of problems, such as depression or anxiety or other changes in behaviors? It is important to ask about their perceptions of their child's current eating pattern. Often the therapist finds that the parents portray a much more disturbed pattern of eating than the patient herself describes. The parents also should provide a general picture of their child's emotional and physical development as a clue to temperamental variables, and family problems and family weight and shape concerns should be identified.

Other Aspects of an Initial Evaluation

In addition to interviewing the patient and family, a medical and nutritional assessment must be conducted. These are important both because they help to confirm the diagnosis and because the therapist needs to know how severely malnourished the child is and what her medical condition will be if she continues to deteriorate. If the therapist does not have a good understanding of basic nutrition and its effects on health, consultation with a dietitian who has expertise in working with eating disorders may be helpful. These trained professionals can help clinicians to determine the patient's current percentage of ideal body weight. An initial goal for most patients with AN is the restoration of physical health. A series of weight goals may be calculated for each patient. This is best done by a nutritionist with experience in the evaluation of patients with eating disorders. The body mass index—weight (kg)/height (m)— is a more precise estimate of healthy targets. Although we believe this type of approach is needed for hospitalized patients, as will become clearer, in our outpatient treatment we focus on using the body's response to nutrition rather than a weight goal per se. For girls this means nutritional rehabilitation that leads to normal menstruation as our goal rather than a specific weight. In the therapy described in this manual, it is assumed that the therapist has access to this type of information and that the adolescent has a trained pediatrician who understands the signs of severe malnutrition.

Medical Evaluation and Treatment

A therapist should be careful to ensure that any patient with AN whom they treat has adequate medical treatment and monitoring. Therapists as a rule should not take responsibility for this aspect of an evaluation or treatment. However, the therapist should be aware of the kinds of assessments that a pediatrician or adolescent medicine specialist might make. In our center, a basic medical workup for an adolescent with AN would include a complete physical to check for signs of malnutrition (e.g., dehydration, tooth erosion, lanugo), as well as tests for liver, kidney, and thyroid functioning. These examinations help to assess the degree of illness and its chronicity, as well as to rule out other possible organic reasons for weight loss, including such things as diabetes, thyroid disease, or cancers (see Table 3.1).

    At times the clinician who is conducting an evaluation becomes

TABLE 3.1. Medical Evaluation

Complete physical

Check for evidence of the following:

- Dehydration
- Orthostasis
- Bradycardia
- Hypothermia
- Physical signs of severe malnutrition (skin changes, lanugo)
- Esophageal tears
- Tooth erosion
- Weight and height

Laboratory tests

- Complete blood count
- Electrocardiogram, electrolytes
- Blood urea nitrogen
- Creatinine
- Thyroid studies
- Urine specific gravity

concerned about the immediate physical health of the adolescent. In fact, at any time during an evaluation or treatment, the need for an acute medical hospitalization may arise. The publication of medical treatment guidelines by the Society for Adolescent Medicine provides consistent patterns of acute hospitalization for adolescents with AN (Society for Adolescent Medicine, 1995). The medical guidelines suggested for hospitalization for patient safety used in this manual are based on those guidelines (see Table 3.2).

TABLE 3.2. Admission Criteria for Acute Hospitalization for Anorexia Nervosa among Adolescents (Lucile Salter Packard Children's Hospital at Stanford University)

- Urine specific gravity > 1.030 or < 1.010
- Pulse rate less than 50 beats/minute
- Orthostatic pulse change: Systolic > 10mmHg or pulse change > 35 beats/minute
- Irregular pulse, QTc > .43
- Syncope
- Temperature < 36.3° C
- Abnormal electrolytes
- Physical examination consistent with dehydration
- < 75% ideal body weight (female)
- Low weight as assessed (male)
- Growth arrest
- Pubertal delay

Standardized Instruments

In addition to the usual clinical interviews, it may be helpful to mention that there are a number of standardized interviews and questionnaires that are sometimes used in the evaluation of children with eating disorders. Specific structured interviews are available in both adult and child versions (Cooper & Fairburn, 1987; Lask & Bryant-Waugh, 1992), and screening instruments can be obtained in parent and child versions (Slade et al., 1990). Clinical self-reports are also available. For example, the Eating Disorder Inventory (EDI) has normative data down to age 14 years (Shore & Porter, 1990). The Eating Attitudes Test (EAT) has a version applicable to school-age children (Maloney et al., 1988), the Kids Eating Disorder Survey to middle-school children (Childress et al., 1993). Some of these instruments may be used in conjunction with clinical interviews as a way of exploring treatment response.

Case Formulation

At the conclusion of the evaluation, the therapist should be comfortable that the patient has a diagnosis of AN and should have some idea about how the family may be structured, which will be further assessed as treatment progresses. Using a manual does not provide all the answers to how to think about a particular family. It does provide a schedule of interventions that apply to all families that enroll in such treatment. Still, there are particular difficulties each family presents that are important for therapists to understand and think about as they implement each strategy. In the following examples, we hope to illustrate some common family structures and issues that therapists may encounter and how we believe the therapeutic maneuvers described in the manual can be used in such situations.

Single-Child Family

The problems in applying this therapy in such a family are that the patient can feel unsupported because she has no sibling allies. As mentioned before, it is helpful if the adolescent has some peer support, but often this is not available and unrelated peers are not included in family sessions. Thus the burden is on the therapist to take up an even more supportive role than would be the case if there were siblings present. This is challenging, especially at the beginning of therapy, when the emphasis is on engaging the parents in active refeeding. On the other hand, because the family is small, there is more time for the therapist to focus on the adolescent. Thus, in small families, it is important for the therapist to manage an appropriate balance between the parents and child that ensures that all feel supported.

Single-Parent Family

This is a corollary situation to the single-child family because in these families the therapist may be an especially important resource to the parent who is without a partner in dealing with this formidable illness. In these cases, the therapist must be careful not to take up the partnership role but should acknowledge that the single parent does not have the same resources as does a couple when negotiating and caring for an ill child. In addition to suggesting that the parent find an additional adult ally (e.g., a grandparent, aunt, uncle, etc.) if one is appropriate and available, the therapist should be prepared to face the reality that she or he will likely be needed more than in two-parent families.

To empower a single parent is complicated. Throughout the refeeding process the therapist should take great pains to make sure that the patient's siblings do not take up a parental role. Instead, the siblings should provide uncritical support and sympathy for the patient. This is a difficult process and one reason why the presence of the siblings in therapy is strongly encouraged. On the other hand, the single parent does not have to negotiate or struggle with disagreements with partners.

One-Distant-Parent Family

Unlike the situation described in single-parent families, the therapist here faces not so much a lack of resources as inaccessible resources. Reasons for one parent being distant can be many. Among the most common are anger at the patient and the illness, preoccupation with self or career, disorganization, problems with the partner, and feelings of incompetence in helping with the illness. Often the distant parent is the father, who has "delegated" the family to the mother. It is important for the therapist to understand the reason for the distance these parents have taken and to have some hypothesis as to why they have removed themselves from the family. The therapeutic maneuver of engaging the parental dyad to take action does not change, but how the therapist accomplishes this may vary. It the parent is actively angry, the therapist needs to find ways to help the parent not to be critical of the child, even while he or she is struggling with these feelings. The seriousness of the illness and the need to take action must be emphasized when confronting parents who are preoccupied or disorganized. Feelings of incompetence are best confronted with available evidence of good parenting.

Sibling in Parental Role

Sometimes when a parent removes himself or herself from the situation of taking care of the child with AN, a sibling may step in to take up the role. As we have suggested from the outset, it is important that parents work together as a parental dyad to combat the illness and that the siblings work at supporting their affected sibling. When a sibling takes over the role of "parent," it causes problems, because it potentially relieves the parent who is not active of the obligation to be engaged in the treatment. It also removes a source of support from the affected child. Hence, when the therapist sees this configuration, it is important that he or she make an effort to redirect the sibling to other, more appropriate, roles. For example, one girl had been monitoring her sister's caloric intake and reporting it to her mother. The therapist suggested that this was a lot of work for her and that it probably had led to conflicts with her sister—which indeed it had. With assistance, the girl identified other, more supportive, ways she could help her sister, including talking to her sister and offering to share foods her sister particularly liked with her.

Patient in Parental Role

There are instances in which the patient has assumed such a dominant role in the family that she or he can be viewed as having taken on similar authority to a parent. Often this is due to the powerful intimidating influence of AN in some family constructs. In such cases, parents may try to avoid confronting AN out of fear they will make matters worse; of course, this generally only increases the impact of the illness on the family by disempowering the parents. In such cases, AN can be said to be "running the family." The therapeutic approach described in this manual applies quite directly to these cases. However, when the pattern of disaffection, avoidance, and inaction on the part of parents has continued for a prolonged period, it will likely take an even greater effort on the part of the therapist to stir the parents to action.

No One in Parental Role

In some families, there appears to be no one willing or able to take up the authority of the parental role. With the advent of AN, the need for parents to take up this role is great, but the task may be perceived as overwhelming to parents who have taken the role of "friend" or "collaborator" to their child rather than of a figure with authority. In these cases, the anorexic child has generally had a history of pseudoindependent behaviors—managing most personal decisions since early childhood—while the parents have been preoccupied with their own careers or emotional lives. These families are particularly challenging because there is little the therapist has to refer the parents to as a record of parenting ability. In order to apply the strategies suggested in this manual, the therapist will need to help the parents "develop" their parenting abilities for the first time, which may be indeed an awesome task. The therapist should expect to provide more direction in these cases than in other family structures.

How Personality Disorders or Personality Disorder Traits Affect Treatment

Although personality disorders are not diagnosed in children and adolescents, clear patterns that are likely to be enduring may have evolved by age 18. These personality variables have been seen to play a role in predicting recovery (Casper et al., 1992). Management of personality disorders per se is again beyond the scope of this manual. Nonetheless, the therapist will undoubtedly need to respond to a variety of personality types among the adolescent patients treated. Some will be avoidant and anxious, others more histrionic and borderline, a few may even have antisocial characteristics. The therapist needs to adjust his or her work and the ways in which support and guidance are offered in response to these variations. Some thoughts about how this might affect treatment follow below.

Avoidant and Anxious Patients

These are the most common types of personality traits likely to be found among pure anorexic patients. The difficulty for the therapist with these patients is to find ways to keep the patient's anxiety and tendency to withdraw from removing her from family therapy. The therapist will likely need to be more actively supportive without being intrusive, while also looking to resources within the family to help. The danger is that the patient will attempt to stay "removed" from the therapy and therefore not benefit.

Histrionic and Borderline Patients

These personality traits are often associated with bulimia nervosa, but some adolescent patients with AN with binge/purge characteristics also share these qualities. These patients are also anxious, but they manage their anxiety by becoming self-destructive and affectively labile and by constantly testing therapeutic boundaries. These types of behaviors are challenging even without disordered eating, but with the added medical and psychological problems of AN, these types of personalities become more hazardous. The therapist who is treating such a patient must pay special attention to attempts by the patient to coopt the therapist. In other words, the patient may attempt to turn family therapy into individual therapy. She may also attempt to split the treatment team. It may be more difficult for the therapist to keep a focus on the disordered eating when self-harming behaviors may seem pressing or other problems more important. The therapist must be alert to all of these possibilities and be prepared to address them, then go back to the main issue at hand. Often such patients have families that are less organized or available to them, and this may make family therapy more challenging.

Setting Up Treatment

It may seem unusual to make special mention of the initial telephone contact. However, this manualized treatment is designed to be time limited, and success depends to a large extent on the therapist's ability to make a powerful connection with the family. Given the formidable task at hand, these initial telephone contacts are crucial for the successful outcome of this process. It is therefore essential that the therapist him- or herself set up the first face-to-face meeting by contacting the family once a referral has been received. From the onset of treatment, which in fact commences with the initial telephone contact, the therapist adopts a grave and concerned tone in order to convey the seriousness of the illness to the family. It may be useful for the therapist, even at this early point, to acknowledge that the parents are demoralized and therefore skeptical of their capacity to do anything. The therapist should help them to see that ensuring that the entire family is present for family therapy is a first step they can take to change these feelings.

The therapist should achieve two aims with the phone contacts to set up the initial family meeting:

1. Establish that there is a crisis in the family and begin the process of defining and enhancing parental authority to manage the crisis.
2. Explain the context of treatment, that is, the treatment team and medical monitoring.

The therapist's first goal is to have every family member attend the sessions. The theoretical rationale for having all family members present is to aid in the therapist's assessment of the family, as well as to maximize the opportunity to help the family; the family plays a role in both the maintenance and the resolution of the eating disorder (Eisler et al., 1997; Le Grange, 1993; Le Grange et al., 1992; Minuchin et al., 1975; Russell et al., 1987; Selvini Palazzoli, 1974). If everyone is not present, the therapist risks losing both power and information. Next the therapist must start to enhance the parental authority even at this very early stage of treatment. This is to strengthen the parents' resolve in making sure that all family members attend the treatment sessions and to begin to prepare them for the task of refeeding their offspring. The process of enhancing parental authority is in accordance with Minuchin's suggestions about defining and clarifying hierarchical structures. From the perspective of structural therapists, strengthening parental authority while aligning the patient with her sibling subsystem enhances hierarchical definition and sets up healthy intergenerational boundaries. This clearer definition should enable the parents to embark on the refeeding task. Both these notions derive from the work of the Philadelphia Child Guidance Clinic (Minuchin et al., 1975; Selvini Palazzoli, 1974). The tone and quality of therapist's communications should take are suggested by the work of Haley (1973) and Madanes' (1981). The tone adopted by the therapist in this therapy is important for a specific reason. The therapist conveys the seriousness of their daughter's illness to the family in a warm and portentous manner both to raise their anxiety and to engage them in treatment.

How the Therapist Achieves These Aims

The therapist must decide beforehand whom to meet at the first face-to-face session, taking the context of treatment into account. Most often the therapist will use the initial telephone contacts to emphasize that there is a crisis in the family (but not one of their making); that is, that their adolescent offspring is starving, that they as a family should respond to this crisis, and that the therapist wants the help of all family members who share a household with the anorexic patient in this matter. Although this is a straightforward arrangement in most instances, it may also require some firmness and tact.

Consequently, the therapist begins by putting forward a convincing request that all those living in the same household should attend. The therapist might say something like the following: "You are the people with the biggest investment of love and commitment to your daughter, so you are also the ones most likely to help the most with this problem." Despite alternative suggestions by family members, the therapist should insist that a whole-family consultation is the only way to address the grave family dilemma. Therefore, this meeting will include the parents and their children, even adult children who may be in full-time employment. In addition, any extended family member, such as a grandparent, uncle, or aunt, who may be living in the same household should be included in this meeting. If the grandparents are not living with the patient and her family, but the patient spends a significant amount of time with them (e.g., if the patient spends several hours per day with her grandparents after school and before her parents return from work), then the therapist may want to include these relatives in treatment as well.

Separated, divorced, or single-parent families may need special arrangements. At first, the custodial parent and his or her household will have to be seen. However, if the patient spends significant amounts of time with the other biological parent, then that parent and his or her household (the secondary household) will need to be incorporated into treatment at some later stage. The nonbiological parents/partners should not experience this arrangement as reconvening the former marriages but rather as an attempt at developing cooperative parenting skills.

These arrangements may seem confusing, but one way to proceed is for the therapist to determine after the initial assessment who is the primary family or household responsible for the refeeding process. This is especially true for parents with shared custody and in cases in which the patient spends an equal amount of time with both parents. Such a decision should be made with the utmost sensitivity, and the therapist should take great pains to communicate to the families that the decision is based on the families' time and resources and that it is not to be taken as a judgment of their ability.

Confirmation Letter

Finally, to demonstrate the seriousness the therapist attaches to the patient's illness, he or she should convey the central therapeutic message to the parents in a detailed letter to the family prior to the first face-to-face meeting (see Figure 3.1). This letter should once more emphasize the seriousness with which the therapist views the patient's illness and how important it is for the entire family to attend this initial meeting. A follow-up call the evening prior to the appointment by the therapist to remind the family of the upcoming meeting will greatly enhance at-

Dear Mr. and Mrs. Smith,

It was a pleasure speaking with you on the telephone to arrange for the first appointment for your family to begin family therapy to assist you with your daughter, who is suffering from anorexia nervosa. I want to emphasize how concerned I am about your daughter's health and how important I believe you and your family can be in helping her to recover. As you know, Anorexia Nervosa is a very serious illness with the highest mortality rate of any psychiatric illness. It is also clear that the earlier and more aggressively we all intervene to help your daughter, the more likely it is that she will return to health.

It is so important that all of your family attend the family therapy. My experience is that everyone in the family has to some degree been affected by anorexia nervosa. It is also my opinion that every family member has something to contribute to the defeat of this illness's hold on your daughter and your family. For these reasons, as we discussed, I require all family members to be present, even though it may be inconvenient for them and may require them to miss other important activities. Your daughter's extreme fragility and need for this treatment requires that all family members make a commitment to her recovery.

Our meeting is scheduled to occur at 3:30 P.M. in my office. Please plan to arrive a few minutes early so that I may weigh your daughter prior to beginning our family meeting.

I very much look forward to assisting you in helping your daughter recover from anorexia nervosa. I am planning to meet with each family member and involve them in your daughter's recovery.

    Yours sincerely,

FIGURE 3.1. Sample letter confirming initial appointment.

tendance. This call will also emphasize the seriousness that the therapist feels for the problem at hand.

Common Difficulties in Setting Up Treatment

What do you do if parents say that it will be impossible for everyone to attend?

The therapist should reinforce appropriate parental authority in order to support the parents to convince everyone in the household to attend. The therapist can begin by saying: "In my experience of this difficult problem, I have always found it best to meet all family members and learn how they view the difficulties, and it is important that you insist that everyone attend." That is, the therapist should impress upon the parents that they have a terrible crisis on their hands and that meeting everyone who lives with the patient and getting an idea from each and every one about their daughter's or relative's illness is essential and extremely valuable information. Impress upon the parents that surely they can convince their children and other household members that their sister or relative is gravely ill and that their opinions are valuable and very helpful in working out a treatment plan. The therapist may say something like: "Although it may seem inconvenient for other family members to attend a family session, your other children will be interested in getting their sister back from anorexia nervosa."

What do you do when nonbiological parents or the patient's secondary household prefer not to participate in treatment?

Similar to convincing the parents that the entire household would be helpful in supporting the therapist in his or her efforts to understand the patient's dilemma, the therapist should first stress that this is not an attempt to reconvene the previous relationship between the biological parents. The therapist should also impress upon all concerned that their participation would be helpful in the swift recovery of the anorexic youngster.

What if parents ask about the "underlying psychological problems" giving rise to AN?

It must be emphasized that in the starved state, the adolescent with AN is not in a position to explore or address these types of issues. They must wait until reasonable progress in weight and nutritional restoration have occurred. These are the types of issues that can and will be addressed in the second and third phases of treatment.

What if the patient presents with another primary disorder (e.g., anxiety, depression, obsessive–compulsive disorder)?

Although the therapist should take care to address any distress the patient may suffer due to a comorbid illness such as depression or anxiety, especially if symptoms are experienced as debilitating, this should in no way become the primary focus of treatment at this stage. Many of these symptoms could be associated with the eating disorder, whereas for some patients it may be a primary diagnosis that predates the onset of their eating disorder. The therapist should note, though, that helping the parents to master the task of refeeding their adolescent offspring may at the same time provide them with the authority and ability to address or contain some of the patient's concomitant psychopathology (i.e., the side effects of starvation). If symptoms persist, the therapist may have someone with expertise in pharmacotherapy join the team, or, if he or she is medically licensed, take on this task him- or herself. Otherwise, the therapist may wish to treat these conditions independently of this manual.

Summary

If these preliminary arrangements have gone well, the likelihood that the first session will also go well is substantially increased. This is the main reason for undertaking them. The telephone call and letter serve as reminders and opportunities to reinforce for the parents the need for action to stop their child from starving and to encourage full participation by the family. In addition, as discussed in Chapter 2, setting up a treatment team serves the purpose of supporting the therapist in his or her activities. In order to be successful, the therapist needs to feel that there is sufficient medical support should the patient not respond to treatment. The therapist also benefits from the support of another clinician as he or she struggles with the realities of getting the therapy started.

4

Session 1: The First Face-to-Face Meeting

The first face-to-face meeting with the family is critical because it sets the tone for the entire first phase of therapy. The therapist has prepared the family through the initial telephone and written contacts that are designed to communicate the importance of everyone's presence and the seriousness of the therapy that the family is about to engage in.

There are three main goals for Session 1:

- To engage the family in the therapy.
- To obtain a history of how the AN is affecting the family.
- To obtain preliminary information about how the family functions (i.e., coalitions, authority structure, conflicts).

In order to accomplish these main goals, the therapist undertakes the following therapeutic interventions:

1. Weighing the patient.
2. Greeting the family in a sincere but grave manner.
3. Taking a history that engages each family member in the process.
4. Separating the illness from the patient.
5. Orchestrating an intense scene concerning the seriousness of the illness and difficulty in recovering.

6. Charging the parents with the task of refeeding.
7. Preparing for next session's family meal and ending the session.

The main strategy is to engage the family about the seriousness of their daughter's condition in a manner that can be described as sympathetic, grave, portentous, and warm. The aim is to raise parental anxiety and concern so that they can take appropriate action, while at the same time reducing parental guilt. It is also critically important to engage the patient in a sympathetic way because of her perceptions of what her parents will be putting her through in the refeeding process. The style in which the therapist engages the family is complex in that the therapist is the deliverer of bad news (e.g., "your daughter is desperately ill and something very drastic has to happen for you to save her life"), while at the same time he or she is also the kind and concerned caregiver who communicates his or her concern in a warm and caring tone (e.g., "you must be devastated and worn out by this terrible ordeal, and not knowing which way to turn to make things better for your daughter must play on your minds all the time"). The therapist should specifically contradict the idea that the family causes AN.

This complex style, also referred to as a therapeutic paradox, is what is believed to be at the heart of engaging the family in treatment. In this session, the therapist will attempt to engage the family in treatment by setting up the therapeutic bind. The therapeutic bind is created by the therapist's authoritative stance toward the parents and the illness on the one hand (i.e., taking charge, being knowledgeable about the illness and what needs to be done to reverse its course) and his or her warmth and acceptance toward the family on the other (i.e., showing sorrow for the state the patient is in and how terribly difficult this must be for everyone). The therapist should succeed in raising the parents' anxiety by acknowledging that they are desperate that something should be done about their daughter's weight and that *they* should do it. Although they may be apprehensive about this task, the therapist's kindness and knowledge about how to get out of this dilemma spurs them on to remain engaged and get on with the job at hand. It is this dichotomy in style, or the therapeutic bind, that should help the family to engage with the therapist in treatment. Put another way, the therapist aims to disorient the family by raising their anxiety while being kind at the same time. This disorientation frees them from their usual patterns and allows them to take the therapist's lead and experiment with new patterns of behavior.

Weighing the Patient

Prior to beginning the family session, the therapist must weigh the patient.

Why

Weighing the patient does not just serve an instrumental goal, it also strengthens the relationship between therapist and patient by helping the patient through a potentially stressful process. The therapist communicates his or her understanding of this difficult process to the patient and so strengthens his or her relationship with the patient. The therapist is therefore able to use both the patient's weight and the relationship aspects that emerge from this process in the family therapy sessions.

How

The therapist should be at hand to monitor the patient's response to any weight change and to address her response to these changes. The patient should be greeted, separated from her family, and asked to join the therapist. As they walk to the weighing-in area, the therapist should ask if the patient has any particular concerns or problems that should be discussed during the upcoming session. In future sessions, this process will be repeated and should become the expected routine opportunity for the patient and the therapist to have a few minutes apart from the family as a whole to allow communication of issues the adolescent may have difficulty bringing forward without the support of the therapist.

The therapist should record the patient's weight on a weight chart, and this information should be conveyed to the family. We recommend that the weight chart be plotted in the presence of the family (Figure 4.1). In this way, the patient's weekly weight will help determine the direction each treatment session will take; if her weight has gone up, the therapist will use this information to congratulate the parents on their efforts and reinforce a continuation of this success. Should the patient's weight stay at a low level or drop, the therapist should use this information to reinvigorate the parent's efforts to refeed their youngster. In addition, the family should be provided with a copy of the weight chart at every session. This should serve as another visual reminder of their daughter's progress (or lack thereof) in regaining her lost weight over time. Because many patients with AN become overly fixated on specific weights or numbers, it is not helpful

Weight Change Per Session

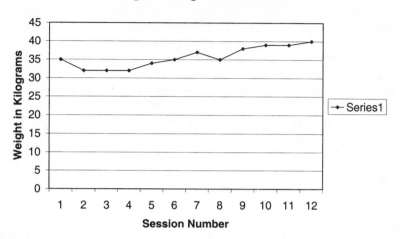

FIGURE 4.1. Example of a weight chart used in therapy sessions.

to focus on specific weight targets in this therapy. Instead, the emphasis should be on the direction of weight gain or loss, and return of menses in young women.

Greeting the Family in a Sincere But Grave Manner

Why

Engaging eating-disordered patients and their families in treatment is often a profound challenge, and the outcome of treatment is affected by the degree to which the therapist succeeds in this task. To emphasize the seriousness of the illness, the style in which the therapist conducts the first greeting—intensely, gravely, empathetically, warmly, sincerely, and with foreboding—is most important. The therapist must make sure that he or she meets each family member, gets to know what he or she does, whether it is work or school related, and check that each family member knows why the family is attending. The therapist should treat every member of the family with the same degree of respect and should make special efforts to let everyone feel that their presence at the meeting is valued.

The successful implementation of this maneuver is totally in the hands of the therapist. The therapist could fail in his or her task if he or she does not sufficiently embrace the family or show elaborate concern for the family's struggle. The cause of such failure could be on unconscious dislike of the family or perhaps frustration because they showed up without all members present. Other causes could include a belief that the family did indeed cause the illness or that the patient or family is intrinsically manipulative, aggressive, or controlling. To combat these problems, the therapist should carefully address these issues with a colleague or cotherapist. The therapist must be able to effectively generate sufficient warmth and concern for the family and their dilemma in order to perform this therapy with success.

How

The therapist invites the family into the room and greets each family member by a handshake or clear eye contact. The therapist is serious and conveys this attitude through facial expression, tone of voice, and calm demeanor. Each family is asked to take a seat of their choosing. Sometimes it is difficult for the therapist to focus adequately on each family member. There may be a tendency to spend more time on the parents at the expense of the patient and siblings. This problem may arise in part because the therapist is aware that the need to stir the parents to action toward the end of the session is paramount and is therefore preparing for this. However, not focusing adequately on each family member would be an error, because at the beginning of the session the entire family needs to be engaged, as they are all needed in the process of helping with recovery. It may help if the therapist reminds families at the beginning of the session that he or she needs to speak to each family member. Then if the therapist must interrupt someone to ensure that other perspectives are heard, the family has been prepared for this. At the same time, it should be remembered that there will be future sessions in which additional information can be gained from each family member, so that if, when reviewing a session, the therapist notes an imbalance in perspectives, this problem can be addressed subsequently.

Taking a History That Engages Each Family Member in the Process

Why

The therapist now turns to the way in which the family members view the eating problem. The therapist should get a detailed description from each family member, including the patient, of how each perceives the anorexic member's state of ill health. The therapist has to succeed in this task so that he or she can highlight the harmful effects of the illness and set the stage for orchestrating an intense scene regarding the patient's illness. The therapist uses a circular style of questioning in order to engage the whole family and to help guard against a single family member or only a few members taking over the session. The purpose of this history taking is not just to gather more information but also to enlighten family members among themselves about how the illness is affecting them. In this sense, it is not so much about history as it is about what is happening to the family currently, which is the result of things that have happened in the past as a result of AN. This information is critical to the therapist as he or she prepares for the other interventions of this session that depend on some knowledge of the impact of AN on the family.

In the process of taking this history, the therapist is likely to discover that the parents or siblings harbor feelings of guilt and blame. Sometimes this happens because they have read about AN and believe that families "cause" the illness. Other times they may have tried to force their daughter to eat and ended up feeling ineffective and angry. This frustration may express itself in anger and hostility toward the daughter. The perspective of this family therapy is that families are not the cause of the illness, or, rather, that the cause of AN is unknown. More important, though, because families are seen as the major resource for helping the adolescent recover, any impediments to this purpose need to be addressed, and guilt is one of them. Unlike anxiety, which we see as motivating parents to take action, guilt tends to cause hesitancy, self-doubt, and ineffectiveness. We therefore spend time in the first session (and in subsequent sessions when the issue comes up again) directly addressing the problem of guilt in order to reduce its impact on parental action in taking charge of refeeding their daughter.

How

Circular questioning is often very helpful in getting an idea from each family member of how they experience the illness; that is, instead of asking the father or the mother how much they worry about their daughter not eating, the therapist can ask the patient or one of the siblings this question. For example, turning to a sibling, the therapist may say, "How do you know that Mom is worried?" and "How can you tell Dad is worried?" Similarly, he or she may ask Mother, "What does your husband do when your daughter struggles to eat?" or ask Dad, "What does your wife typically do to encourage your daughter to eat more?" The way in which each family member describes the problem influences the therapist's response to the family. The therapist reflects the family's comments back to them in such a way as to amplify the seriousness of the problem and the family's sense of having done all it could do to help without success. The therapist may end up saying, "So, what I hear from you is that you and many others have tried so hard to help your daughter to recover from this dreadful illness, and still the illness had clawed its way back. In fact, it has overtaken your daughter's life completely, so much so that she is dying unless we can succeed in nourishing her back to health." Although the content of the therapist's words should concentrate on the horror of this life-threatening illness, the tone should still be as warm, friendly, and positive about the family as possible.

It is also important to spend some time on a direct discussion of "who's to blame for the AN," the aim of this intervention being to dispel and contradict existing belief about this. It is also important that the therapist spend time addressing the patient, specifically in terms of acknowledging her current skills, her power, and her achievements. Again, the successful conclusion of this maneuver depends on the therapist's ability to get a sufficiently detailed history from the family.

Separating the Illness from the Patient

Why

In stressing that the patient has little control over her illness, the therapist tries to enable the parents to take drastic action against the illness and not against their daughter, when ordinarily they might be reticent to "force food" onto such an obviously frail-looking adolescent. Therefore, it is important that the therapist model his or her support of the patient who has been "overtaken" by this illness. All of the information about how devastating the illness is and how the parents have to work hard at combating its effects may perturb the patient, and she may fear that the therapist is exaggerating the problem. She may also fear that she is not being understood and that the therapist is about to unleash the family on her, the latter of which is true. This is an important challenge for the therapist, who has to show the patient that although her dilemma is understood, at the same time she needs to gain weight, which is the exact opposite of her wishes. By stressing that AN is not identical to the patient herself, the therapist can emphasize the support for the developing adolescent, while at the same time distinguishing AN as a problem the patient has. This strategy is key in maintaining engagement with the adolescent while attacking AN. Failure to achieve this separation can increase resistance to the treatment on the patient's part.

While going through the process of separating the illness from the patient, the therapist may find that family members respond to some of the patient's comments about food and weight by being critical of her. It is important from the outset that a noncritical stance toward the patient or her symptoms be modeled for the family by the therapist, and this separation of AN from the patient is an excellent first opportunity.

Modeling uncritical acceptance of the patient is an essential therapeutic task for the therapist, as the therapist must succeed in externalizing the illness, that is, refusing to identify the patient with the illness. Research on expressed emotion has shown that parental criticism toward the patient contributes to early dropout from treatment (Le Grange, Eisler, Dare, & Hodes, 1992). In addition, high levels of parental criticism and hostility toward the patient exacerbate the eating-disorder symptoms and have negative impact on treatment outcome. We have found that many families with an anorexic youngster are very reluctant to express any criticism of their child. However, in this situation, even low levels of criticism (i.e., two to three critical comments of the patient counted in a 1-hour treatment session) can lead to an increase in eating-disorder symptomatology, an increase in parents' criticism of their child, and consequent poor treatment progress. Therefore, by modeling uncritical acceptance of the patient and her symptoms (i.e., showing the parents that most "illness behavior" is not within the patient's control), the therapist will foster an understanding of the patient's behavior and reduce any parental criticism of her. It is helpful to specifically say that a noncritical attitude is not "normal" in most families but is therapeutically essential: "Sometimes parents have to do unusual things to save their child's life." It may be useful to provide an analogy of the efforts required of parents who have to do such "unusual things," such as offering their organs for transplantation or providing unusual amounts of custodial care (e.g., for children with cystic fibrosis).

How

The therapist should ask the patient to list all the things the illness has given her, as well as taken away from her. As he or she listens to this list, the therapist must show as much warmth for the patient and as much distress and fear about the symptoms as possible and may say: "I am saddened that this terrible illness has interrupted your life to this degree, that it has taken your freedom away, and that it has left you without much control of what you do." In doing this, it is vitally important for the therapist to show not only sympathy for the family but also an understanding of the patient. The therapist must model an un-critical attitude toward the patient's symptoms and must simultaneously show warmth toward the patient and just as much distress and fear about the symptoms and their consequences. He or she may say, "I know that you are more frightened of eating, sometimes, than of dying. Dying seems a long way off, food is right in front of you." It is essential that the therapist attend to and modify any parental and sibling criticism of the patient. The therapist may point out, "The symptoms don't belong to your daughter; rather, it is this terrible illness that has overtaken her and is determining almost all of her activities. For instance, it is AN that makes her hide food, or dispose of food, or makes her behave in deceitful ways. In other words, it is the illness that gets your daughter to do all these things that you find so upsetting. The daughter you knew before this illness took over is not in charge of her behavior, and it is your job to strengthen your daughter once more." Consequently, the therapist will model sympathy and understanding of the patient to the parents, especially a totally noncritical attitude toward the patient's symptoms and an understanding that it is the illness that has temporarily halted her development. To support this perspective, the therapist may say: "I do not want for a moment for you to feel that your spirit is broken. I want to help your parents save your life, but not to give them control over anything else."

Orchestrating an Intense Scene Concerning the Seriousness of the Illness and Difficulty in Recovering

Why

Next, the therapist wishes to raise parental anxiety and concern by orchestrating an intense scene concerning the seriousness of AN in order to increase their sense of responsibility to take on a dreadful task at which others have had limited success. In this sense, anxiety is a useful motivator, whereas guilt and blame are not. Successful restoration of their daughter's health through weight gain depends on the parents' unified action in the refeeding process in much the same way as competent and caring nursing staff would act if the patient were admitted to a specialist inpatient unit. The therapist is summarizing his or her findings and is now going to deliver his or her salvo. That is, the therapist should model grieving over the past treatment failures in the context of the present treatment. Although being careful not to discredit previous attempts at restoring the patient's weight, the therapist is taking this step to help demonstrate to the parents that they are indeed their child's last resort. One approach to this is to help the family to explore what did not work in previous therapy. Successfully grieving over past failures is believed to further mobilize the parents in taking drastic action toward weight restoration. At the same time, the theory behind this "drama" is that if the therapist can succeed in reawakening the parents' power and skills in feeding their child, they will be energized to take action and succeed in returning their daughter's health. It is for the parents to get past placation or denial and to embrace their anger and fear about the illness instead. The therapist is therefore "stirring up the family" in order to call on their resources. We do not want the family to even entertain the idea of not taking on this task.

How

The therapist should now orchestrate an intense scene that neither scapegoats the patient, blames the parents, nor exempts the siblings. The foci of this action should be the patient's weight, the failed previous attempts at weight restoration, the medical and emotional problems likely to occur if AN persists, and the emphasis on the point that the family is the last resort for the patient. For example, if the patient has been in the hospital, the therapist should alarm the family about the potential for rapid weight loss. If weight gain in the hospital has been unsatisfactory, he or she should lament that failure. The ineffectiveness of past health care professionals' efforts should be treated respectfully but held out as further evidence of the dire position the family finds themselves in. Regardless of the specifics of each patient and her family, the therapist should impress upon the parents the following: "Most couples have a variety of ways in which they approach everyday issues and dilemmas in their families. You as a couple may also have some issues that you differ on, and that is okay. However, when it comes to working out a plan about how to nourish X back to health, you cannot afford to disagree at all, you have to work together all the time. The slightest disagreement between the two of you will make it easy for the eating disorder to stay in charge of your daughter's life and defeat her. You have to act as if you are one person in order to succeed." Upon gathering information from the family about how they experience the illness, the therapist then tells the family what it is he or she "hears" the family telling them ("reflection") but in such a way as to amplify (increase) the seriousness of the illness. The therapist should be genuine and purposeful in his or her expression of the "horror, despair, panic, and hopelessness of the family." The therapist may find it helpful to show his or her empathy by holding close to the actual medical seriousness of the illness, the patient's corpse-like appearance, and the horror of the illness. It may be helpful for the therapist to think of other non-eating-disordered cases of dying children. To illustrate this concern, the therapist may say something akin to the following: "Your child is dying of this disorder." Also, the therapist must work hard not to accept the AN façade that "everything is all right." Paradoxically, this could very well be a pitfall for experienced therapists, who could be "seduced" by their familiarity with the illness. On the other hand, less experienced therapists may let the horror of the illness overwhelm them and consequently become immobilized. The therapist must try to raise the family's activation energy, as habit, family structure, and patient resistance are all aspects that may inhibit parental ability to take charge of refeeding their daughter.

Charging the Parents with the Task of Refeeding

Why

After the therapist has described the difficulties and failures of past efforts to help the patient and the consequences of inaction, he or she must next help the family to see that no matter what other treatments may be available in the short term, the patient will finally return to the family. This prepares the family for the charge that the therapist is about to make, that they need to refeed their daughter. The family will likely be horrified, angry, or resentful with the therapist's suggestion that they ought to help restore the patient's health. The reasons that the family is the best resource for refeeding their daughter include that they know her best, that they are the most invested in her well-being and future health, that they have shown evidence of being good parents in the past, and that, as an adolescent, their daughter still needs her family.

How

The therapist should now make a case for the family being the major resource for their daughter's recovery. The therapist should first point out what the other treatment alternatives are (e.g., hospitalization, individual therapy, residential treatment) and how they might soon put the family in the same predicament as before, that is, having a severely underweight offspring. Although the therapist should leave the decisions as to how to accomplish the refeeding to the parents, it may help to offer them some ideas to consider, for example, organizing meals so that the parents can monitor them more effectively by having two breakfasts (before school), an early dinner, and a late supper. She or he should also alert the parents not to become engaged in discussions about diet foods and emphasize that they should nourish the patient according to her profound state of malnutrition, not according to the wishes of AN. This therapy is aimed at patients who are medically stable and should require no special dietary advice other than to eat nourishing and fattening foods. It is important that the therapist be able to support the parents' explorations and attempts at refeeding rather than provide them with a prescribed menu, calorie recommendation, or other formulas for recovery. However, the therapist at the same time must not collude with any denial or avoidance of the need to refeed the starving adolescent by allowing to go unchallenged measures that are clearly in the service of AN.

The therapist should press upon the parents that for the first few weeks of treatment it may be necessary for the patient to be absent from school and under parental supervision 24 hours per day. Similarly, the therapist may advise the parents that one or both of them might need to take a leave of absence from work in order to accomplish the task of refeeding.

The therapist is making a case for drastic action on several fronts. For instance, it may not be sufficient to say that the patient has to eat more; in fact, the parents may have to be encouraged to stay home with the patient so that they can do the task they have now been given. The therapist should acknowledge the force of what the parents are saying if they express their bewilderment about the difficult task ahead. The therapist may say: "I realize that you may be horrified thinking that you have come to me for help with your daughter, while I in turn have put the ball back in your court. However, we really don't have any alternatives that can secure your daughter's well-being in the long run. Surely we can try and return her to the hospital [if she was hospitalized], which may even have the desired effect in the short term. Most patients, though, lose weight once they are discharged, and then you have to face the same dilemma once more. If you can do this job yourselves, then you can give your daughter the best guarantee to recover fully."

Preparing for Next Session's Family Meal and Ending the Session

The therapist should end the session with great sympathy and sorrow, but also with a sense of optimism that the parents will be able to work out a way to save their daughter's life. Thus the therapist leaves the family with a sense of responsibility to take on this awesome task of refeeding their daughter. The therapist may say: "I know this may be the toughest thing you have ever done, and I also know that it may go against what you intuitively feel is right. This and the fact that your daughter is so terribly ill must weigh heavily on you. However, taking on this very difficult task is the best way forward right now." He or she will invite the family to return within a few days and ask them to bring a picnic lunch with enough food for the patient and everyone else—not based on the patient's wishes but rather on her level of starvation. In other words, the parents should make a decision as to an appropriate meal to serve their starving offspring.

End-of-Session Review

As should be the case at the end of each treatment session, the lead therapist should communicate with therapy and consultation team members and review the following questions.

Common Questions for Session 1

What if some family members fail to show up for the first session?

The therapist's response will, in part, depend on how closely he or she adheres to a "purist" view of family therapy, that is, subscribing only to whole family therapy or adhering to the view that a family consists of several subsystems that can be seen separately in treatment. Some therapists will make it very clear to the family from the outset that they work with the family only when all members are present and may even decline to interview an "incomplete" family. We would, however, advocate a more accommodating view. The advantage of going ahead with the meeting despite the absence of some family members is that the therapist indicates the urgency to attend to the illness without delay. Given the serious nature of the illness, it may be difficult to have the family return home "empty-handed," and the therapist may choose to interview the patient and all family members who present themselves for the first session. The therapist can then use this first face-to-face session to stress the importance of meeting every member of the patient's household and encourage them to cajole the absent member(s) to attend the next family meeting. The risk in going ahead with meeting an "incomplete" family is twofold. First, the therapist is somewhat hampered in that she or he does not get the opportunity to see the family as a whole and can only make inferences regarding interaction patterns between the present and absent members. This may hinder the therapist in her or his efforts to engage all family members in addressing the patient's eating-disorder symptoms. Second, starting therapy without everyone present may reinforce for those present, as well as for the absentees, that treatment can continue without the absent family members.

What if the patient does not want her family to know her weight?

Some patients may resist the idea that their families know their weights, and the therapist may feel trapped between showing respect for the developing adolescent autonomy on the one hand while doing the work of therapy on the other. One way that this dilemma can be addressed is for the therapist to say, "Although the patient is a young adult in many respects, when it comes to eating and weight, she is like a very young child, and the eating disorder is not allowing her to think rationally about things related to food and weight. It is therefore very important for you as parents to help her out in this regard, that is, until she has regained her weight. For this task it is imperative that we monitor X's weight and check it together each session." Turning to the patient, the therapist may say, "I know this is awful for you, and you must be upset with all of us telling you what to do. I am sorry for that, but while you are so terribly thin, it would be dangerous for me to listen to your anorexia speaking, as this illness would not allow you to get healthy, and we cannot let that happen." This personification of AN is a method of externalizing the illness, that is, separating the patient from the illness.

What if the patient expresses a wish not to be weighed?

Similar to the preceding, the therapist should show his or her understanding for the patient's reluctance to being weighed. However, as weight progress is at the essence of the treatment, especially during Phase I, the therapist takes a firm but gentle stance that there is no way forward unless weight status is checked routinely by the therapist. If this view is stated up front with conviction and compassion and without apology, very few patients resist being weighed.

What if the family resists taking a leave of absence from work?

Some families may initially be resistant to the idea that they may have to take time out of their jobs to make this therapy work. It is, however, very important that the therapist remain adamant in emphasizing that the serious nature of the illness requires drastic steps to rectify. The therapist has to make sure that he or she optimizes the parents' chances at succeeding in this difficult task. Insufficient supervision of the adolescent's eating early on in treatment could lead to a continuation of an environment in which it is possible for the patient to restrict food intake. Therefore, the therapist has to work diligently to persuade the parents that such a drastic step as taking time out of the office is called for under these circumstances. At the same time, the therapist should reassure the parents that this is a temporary step and that there is reason for hope. The therapist may want to evoke analogies with other cases of physical illness for which it is required that parents may have to take time out from work to care for their child, such as cystic fibrosis or cancer.

What if the patient refuses support?

For the patient to refuse either parental or sibling support is not an option. The parents have to set up a meal regimen at home by which eating and completing a meal promptly occur—the expectation for this to occur is relentlessly powerful. In other words, the culture that is created by the parents is that there is no alternative to compliance with eating. This is similar to the culture of the meal regimen that occurs in a well-functioning dedicated eating-disorders unit. If the parents succeed in closing all the loopholes for anorexic behaviors, it would be impossible for the adolescent to be able to refuse support. Setting up such a regimen will require time and patience, and the therapist will have to work hard to review every week exactly how the parents have gone about setting up this regimen. In order to help the patient to understand and empathize with the parents, the therapist may say, "Your parents will want to be able to reassure themselves, if you die from AN, that they have done everything possible to save your life." For further clarification, see Sessions 4 through 12.

What if the siblings are resistant to helping their sister?

Most siblings become horrified to discover that their sister is gravely ill and would like to help if they can. In fact, many siblings might tell you about their previous failed efforts at helping their sister. This is especially true if the premorbid intersibling relationships were sound. However, some siblings may have given up on their ill sister and appear to be resistant in helping any further. As may be the case with the parents, it is imperative that the therapist raises the siblings' concern for their sister and tells them how crucial their helpful behavior will be in restoring their sister's health. The therapist may say, "Brothers and sisters become more and more important as you grow older. You can't afford to lose one." Insisting on their presence at every treatment session is helpful, while making sure that information is gathered from each and every one during treatment sessions will help to make the siblings feel that their presence in the session and assistance at home indeed make a difference to their sister's well-being. It is the principal job of the siblings to support their ill sister through this period and not to make direct efforts to help with refeeding, as refeeding is the parents' task.

5

Session 1 in Action

*T*his chapter provides an example of Session 1. It begins with a short background on the patient and her family. The session is divided into major parts by the interventions. In addition, as the session unfolds, explanatory text guides the reader as to the aims the therapist has in mind.

To review, there are three main goals for Session 1:

- To engage the family in the therapy.
- To obtain a history of how the AN is affecting the family.
- To obtain preliminary information about how the family functions (i.e., coalitions, authority structure, conflicts).

In order to accomplish these main goals, the therapist undertakes the following therapeutic interventions:

1. Weighing the patient.
2. Greeting the family in a sincere but grave manner.
3. Taking a history that engages each family member in the process.
4. Separating the illness from the patient.
5. Orchestrating an intense scene concerning the seriousness of the illness and difficulty in recovering.
6. Charging the parents with the task of refeeding.
7. Preparing for next session's family meal and ending the session.

Clinical Background

Susan is a 17-year-old woman who was diagnosed with AN approximately 6 months prior to the beginning of family therapy. She had been hospitalized for about 3 weeks for severe malnutrition and medical instability approximately 6 weeks prior to beginning family therapy. Although her major strategy for weight loss was caloric restriction, she also engaged in occasional binge-eating and purging behaviors. She is the third child and the only daughter of five children. Her two older brothers are living outside the home. Her two younger brothers (Dan, 10, and Paul, 12) are the products of her mother's second marriage. Susan is their half sister. Susan's mother worked full-time during most of Susan's childhood. Susan has at times filled the role of substitute mother for her two youngest brothers. Susan began family therapy because she has continued to lose weight since her discharge from the hospital and the family is worried about her needing to be readmitted.

Weighing the Patient

Prior to beginning the session, the therapist takes Susan to be weighed. During this process, he discusses with her briefly her feelings about beginning therapy. She is noncommittal but says she will try.

Greeting the Family in a Sincere but Grave Manner

The therapist looks each family member in the eyes and shakes their hands warmly as each of them enters the room. He aims to appear both serious and welcoming.

THERAPIST: Please take any seat over here. I'd like to start by getting each of you to introduce yourselves and tell me a little bit about you.
    (*Nervous laughter from all family members*)

MOTHER: Gee, don't go all at once. Well, I guess, umm, I get to be the mother, and these are three of my five children. There's two older boys. And, umm, I work full time as a manager.

THERAPIST: (*warmly*) That's a good start.

FATHER: Well, I'm Tom. I'm the newest guy on the block here . . . and I just got married 2 years ago in February. So I am their stepfather.

I'm 52. I work as a manager in a large factory. I've been there almost 30 years.

THERAPIST: Okay.

SUSAN: Well, geez, I'm Susan, I'm the reason we're all here. (*laughter*) You probably know everything about me since you have my chart, so. . . .

THERAPIST: Actually I don't, really.

SUSAN: Well, I'm 17, I just turned 17 last week. And . . .

THERAPIST: Happy birthday.

SUSAN: Well, thank you. That's it. That's all I have to say about myself.

PAUL: My name's Paul. I'm in the 7th grade . . . (*laughter*) . . . I don't know.

THERAPIST: What do you like to do?

PAUL: I like to play baseball.

THERAPIST: Anything else?

PAUL: Play football.

THERAPIST: Uh-huh.

DAN: I'm Dan, I'm 10 years old. I'm her sister.
    (*Laughter*)

SUSAN: My sister?
    (*Laughter*)

DAN: Yeah, I'm your sister.

PAUL: You're the brother.

DAN: I'm the brother.

THERAPIST: What grade are you in, Dan?

DAN: Fifth.

THERAPIST: Thank you. Let me tell you why I'm here. I've worked with a lot of young women with eating disorders and hope to help your family.

The therapist's job here is to make everyone feel acknowledged by introducing himself and to give every family member an opportunity to say something about themselves, for example, what they do or what their interests are. In addition, the therapist introduces his authority and competence in order to lay the groundwork for the charge he will make later, which depends on the family recognizing this expertise.

Taking a History That Engages Each Family Member in the Process

Continuing a warm and empathic stance, the therapist further attempts to engage the family by taking a history of the effect of AN on the family to date. Again, the therapist works his way through the family, engaging each in turn with real interest and focus.

THERAPIST: But I'd like to hear a little bit more from all of you about what's going on and how it's going. I'd really like to hear from each of you what this is like for you, dealing with this eating-disorder problem in the family.

FATHER: Well, it's a constant state of worry, concern. We're trying not to stand on top of her, whatever, push her to eat. But by the same token we want to make sure that she is taking in what she is supposed to be taking in. And trying to give her some space, and trying to let her manage it. But it's just kind of difficult because there are times when we're not sure that she's doing what she's supposed to be doing. And then ... so.... The first few days when she was out of the hospital, we thought she was doing extremely well. We were very pleased with what she was doing. And then school started, and it's kind of gone downhill from there.

THERAPIST: You said you were in a constant state of worry?

FATHER: Well, yeah, it seems like since she's started back at school, she's not taking in what she's supposed to be taking in. That's our impression. That's the way it turned out today ... at her clinic visit.

THERAPIST: So that's since the hospitalization. What about even before?

FATHER: Well, before that. When we became aware of it was probably not too much before she was in the hospital. It's been kind of a struggle. For a period of time before that, because she decided, you know she's a vegetarian, and it's been very tough to make sure that she's eating a balanced diet as a vegetarian. But, uh, it seemed like, I don't know, out of the blue, all of a sudden, that she basically stopped eating. We had her to see the doctor a few times before she got admitted to the hospital. And had a visit with a therapist. I guess our lifestyles ... for a while, we were basically bumping into each other in the night. We didn't see a lot of each other. Her mom works a lot of hours. And Susan was involved in sports and schoolwork and everything else. So we were not around each other very much, other than to say hi, I guess. It just kind of snuck up on us.

THERAPIST: (*to Mother*) Did you experience the same kind of worry and fear?

MOTHER: Probably more like panic.

THERAPIST: Uh-huh. . . .

MOTHER: (*crying*) Well, it's this . . . all your life, you love something. And because you love it you take care of it. And you know what you need to do to make it . . . whatever it is, whether it's a stuffed animal, a dog or a cat, you provide for it. And suddenly you have a baby. And you provide for it. And you know everything to do. You know how to change it, and love it, and care for it. And then something like this comes, and you can't fix it. No matter how hard you try. Obviously I do. But you know, she doesn't need changing. I can't fix it. So I feel very frustrated, helpless, angry, guilty.

THERAPIST: Where does the guilt come from? Are there things you think you should have done differently?

MOTHER: Things I should have maybe done differently, I should have maybe been there more.

THERAPIST: What kinds of things have the two of you tried? You said you tried doing things where you don't have to step on toes.

MOTHER: Well, let's see. Before she was hospitalized, I think I tried being supportive, and concerned, and then that didn't work. And then I tried being a bully, and force her to eat. And that didn't work. Since she's been out of the hospital, I've tried to be here, and. . . .

THERAPIST: She's still here.

MOTHER: Barely (*laughing*).

THERAPIST: Well, but she's here. You're doing something right.

The therapist responds to each of the parents' reports by identifying the primary emotional state and gently repeating it so as to amplify the emotional tone. In addition, the therapist wishes to diminish the self-blame and guilt at this point and instead focuses on the positive achievements of the family.

MOTHER: And now, I can't fix it. I can't do anything about it. I can't do anything about it when she feels so unhappy with herself, that she hurts herself, or she takes laxatives, or she does those things. I can't stop it. Because I can't be there 24 hours a day, 7 days a week, wherever she is. I don't know how to help her.

THERAPIST: How has this affected you, Paul?

PAUL: I just probably want it to get over with.

THERAPIST: Why do you want it to get over with? How does it affect you?

PAUL: I don't know, everybody is worried, sad, and stuff.

THERAPIST: Can you say how that makes you feel?

PAUL: It makes me feel sad, and unhappy. I mean, I don't know.

THERAPIST: That's pretty clear to me. How about you, Dan?

DAN: I feel pretty much the same. Because I want her to be home, but I don't want her home now because I don't want her not to be fixed, I don't want her not to be eating. So I want her home but not right now. If I want her home, I want her home fixed and healthy and all right.

THERAPIST: So you're worried, too, and you felt she was safer in the hospital.

DAN: Uh-huh.

THERAPIST: What about you, Susan? You went last this time, it doesn't mean you're last in the equation. What's going on with you about this eating problem? What keeps it going?

SUSAN: Well, I think that I'm doing all right. But, no one else seems to think so. I'm doing better since Monday. I've been purge free since Monday, so that's good. Umm, what's getting me going? My main motivation is to stay out of the hospital, that's the last place I want to be. And to hopefully resume a seminormal life.

THERAPIST: How about a normal life? Is that beyond your hopes for now?

SUSAN: Well, eventually. I don't know how normal it could ever be when your thoughts are always consumed with food. But, maybe with time it will become less of a worry for me. But I'd like to be able to play volleyball again, and to do that I have to get back into my normal exercise routine.

In the preceding exchange, the therapist carefully explores the impact the eating disorder has had on everyone in the family. It is important to get an idea from everyone in order to make an assessment of how AN has affected the family. But asking everyone also helps make every family member feel that his or her opinion counts. The therapist might have employed more "circular" questioning of family members that would allow further commentary and/or elaboration of initial comments.

THERAPIST: Hmm, so, what kinds of things have you tried as a family to help Susan? What kinds of specific things?

MOTHER: Well, we went out and we bought groceries. 'Course, we didn't even buy exactly the kind of groceries that I wanted to, but we did buy groceries.

THERAPIST: You mean the two of you went?

MOTHER: Susan and I went, yeah.

SUSAN: (mumbling)

MOTHER: 'Course she won't eat anything unless it's fat free. Which worries me. We don't exactly agree on that. But, she said she would eat it if we bought it without fat, and if we bought it with fat she wouldn't eat any of it. So, that was kind of fun.

THERAPIST: So you tried shopping together, but it doesn't sound like you feel like it was very successful because you knew she needed fat in her diet. Other things?

FATHER: I've seen a couple things since we've been home from the hospital that I thought Susan did remarkably well. I thought it was a pretty big step, and I think it shouldn't all be negative.

THERAPIST: Sure. Absolutely.

FATHER: In the hospital she said. "I'm not going to eat in front of you." But in the whole first 3 days she was home, 4 days actually, most of the time she ate, she brought it in to wherever we were, and ate it. She hasn't sat at the dinner table with us yet, but last night was close. She actually took food off the dinner table, and ate that, which is a first. So, she's done some remarkably good things, and I felt very positive about that because she was very adamant about not eating around us at all. So, I thought that was some good things that she did, and I was very pleased.

THERAPIST: So there are some good things.

FATHER: And when you see that, of course, it gives you a positive feeling, because you see her eating, and she seems to be making a conscious effort to meet her calorie intake, and so forth.

THERAPIST: Even though she continued to lose weight.

FATHER: She's had a couple bad days. Primarily when she started back at school.

THERAPIST: Do you think it's been only a couple bad days?

MOTHER: Well, Wednesday night when she finally got home at about 8:30. That was a good day.... And Thursday....

THERAPIST: What made it a good day?

MOTHER: She got home from the hospital, that made it a good day. And she pretty much, she was very happy to be home. And she looked really good. And she was excited. And Thursday when we went shopping, even though we didn't agree on what we were going to buy, we still had a good day. We did a lot of things together. She made a conscious effort to eat. That was a good day. Friday was a good day, it seemed like to me. Starting on Saturday, she wasn't doing well. Sunday it got worse.... And Monday was supposed to be the first day back to school, and she was....

SUSAN: I wasn't as worried as you seem to think I was, I really wasn't.

MOTHER: But, she didn't go to school Monday. Sometime on the weekend things started not going so well. Tuesday she went to school. But it sounded like, when I talked to her Tuesday night, that she told me that she had gotten the calories she needed. Yesterday, she didn't go to school, which concerned me. Also because she was by herself. Also because she was missing more school. She did come to lunch with us, so she wasn't by herself the whole entire day.

THERAPIST: She had lunch with you?

MOTHER: We had a fine lunch.

In the preceding exchanges, the therapist tries to balance a need to be supportive of the parents' sense of optimism and hope while not colluding with denial or avoidance of the ongoing evidence of continued problems with disordered eating. Thus the therapist notes the positive achievements but gently reminds the family of the limited success of their interventions to date.

THERAPIST: Dan, you said you were worried about your sister. What are you worried about?

DAN: Well, because I don't want her to go back to the hospital, because she was already there for like 2 months.
  (*Laughter*)

MOTHER: A little less than that, more like a month. It seemed like 2 months. It seemed like a year.

DAN: I don't want her to go back, cause we missed her, so that's what I'm worried about.

THERAPIST: It sounds to me that you were worried that she might have to go back, because she wasn't taking care of herself the way she needs to.

DAN: Not really, I don't really think that she needs to go back, I just don't want her to get sick or anything, because she was sick on Monday and Sunday and all week.

THERAPIST: So you're worried about her? Why are you worried about her being sick? What is it about being sick? Do you think she could die?

DAN: Not really. (*to Susan*) I can hear your stomach

SUSAN: It's not my stomach, it's Tom's. You're not going to be able to hear our voices on the videotape, you're just going to hear Tom's stomach.

THERAPIST: Do you have worries, Paul?

PAUL: I think that she's doing okay, compared to how she was before she went. So I'm just hoping it will get over soon.

The therapist begins to expose the impact that an eating disorder has on the adolescent as well as the family. He works toward preparing the stage to create a scenario to demonstrate to everyone that this is a serious illness and that patients may in fact die as a result of their starvation.

THERAPIST: I guess in the hospital, I don't know if you've talked about it. Just how serious, really, this disease is. Have you talked about that?

PAUL: A little way back.

THERAPIST: What do you remember about it?

PAUL: That umm . . . because I brought Skittles to her once, when she first got in. She gave me a real lecture on it. Then she just talked about it, because she can't do that stuff anymore because of being healthy. (*Laughter*)

THERAPIST: You brought Skittles? Are those candies?

SUSAN: You don't know what Skittles are?

Although toward the end of this exchange, the therapist is more lighthearted, both with the family and the patient, over the Skittles incident, the therapist allows only a brief respite from the intensity of the meeting. The therapist has now gathered everyone's impression of the impact the illness has had on him or her, and in so doing, highlighted the severe impact the eating disorder has already had on the patient. The therapist's task now is to spend some time distinguishing the wishes of Susan from those of AN. In addition to raising the parents' concern about the consequences of the illness, the therapist attempts to give the parents a "handle" on managing the illness. This is done by separating the illness from the adolescent. By saying that the illness "is not part of your daughter," the therapist makes it easier for the parents to understand that the changes they have seen in their daughter have been imposed by the illness. This understanding enables them to take charge of the illness without feeling they are being too up-front or un-democratic in their dealings with their offspring. In this session, sepa-rating the illness from the patient is part of orchestrating the intense scene about the need for action, and these two maneuvers are in fact fairly integrated in this session, as is noted.

Separating the Illness from the Patient

THERAPIST: I'm wondering how much the doctors have told you about how serious anorexia nervosa is? In terms that this is a disease people die from. People die in relatively high rates for a psychiat-ric illness; in fact, it has the highest mortality rate of any psychiat-ric illness. And even if someone doesn't die from the illness, there are many medical problems that also develop as a result of the starvation.

MOTHER: Don't know that they've talked to us about that. . . . It has been related to the inability to bear children later in life. . . .

THERAPIST: That's right, that can happen and is a very serious problem.

FATHER: Kidney damage.

MOTHER: Heart.

FATHER: Heart problems.

THERAPIST: That's right. And emotional problems, like depression. Also, just not ever living up to potential in general, because of always worrying about food and weight. I bring that out because I want ev-eryone to understand why as a family this is something that you all have to really look squarely in the face. It's something that all of you can help with and that all of you are going to need to help with in or-der to help Susan get over this. In some ways this is really very dif-ferent than what you would expect to be doing for a 17-year-old person. Because this disorder is really disrupting her ability to care for herself. That's pretty clear. (*to Susan*) Wouldn't you agree with that too? It's affecting how you take care of yourself.

SUSAN: (*nodding*)

THERAPIST: And putting you (*to Susan*) at risk for all these other problems. Now, I want to make clear, that I'm separating the illness from Susan. Sometimes it may feel like you are the anorexia nervosa. . . .

SUSAN: One and the same.

THERAPIST: Do you feel that way sometimes?

SUSAN: Yeah.

THERAPIST: Can you ever get them apart and see that there are parts of you that really aren't connected with the illness? That part of you that wants to play volleyball, for example?

SUSAN: Yeah.

THERAPIST: That you don't want your brothers worrying that you're going to fall over and have to go back to the hospital. There're parts of you that you can connect to that don't have anything to do with the illness. Because, really, my perspective on it is that it is separate from you. Your illness is really kind of creeping in over you and beginning to cover over who you really are. You can feel the difference. If you really think about it carefully you can sort of see. These parts who are not me, I wouldn't be doing these things if I didn't have this illness. Can you give me some examples. . . .

SUSAN: Umm, let's see. No. If I wasn't ill, I would not hoard food in my bedroom so I can torture myself with not eating it. And I wouldn't bake huge quantities of food just to not eat it. And I would . . . Oh geez, I can name a million things.

THERAPIST: Give me a few more, not a million, but I'm glad you have that list. That's great.

SUSAN: I wouldn't think about, like, how many calories in every food that I eat. And I wouldn't think of ways to burn it off.

THERAPIST: You'd think about other things is what you're saying.

SUSAN: Really, my life would be a little, umm . . . less centered on food.

THERAPIST: You could think about other things?

SUSAN: Yeah, you know, I was just, I turned on the TV, and I was like, oh my gosh, we're like bombing Iraq, and I had no idea. It's like I'm missing all this stuff, and you know, I just really didn't care. I turned on the TV, and was kind of like, whoa, there's like a war almost going on, and I'm missing it, and the world outside is still happening. And I'm in here in my own little sick world.

The therapist now starts to prepare the family for the suggestion that will come toward the end of the session that they will need to refeed their daughter. While doing this, he demonstrates to the patient that he understands her dilemma and models an uncritical stance toward the patient to the rest of the family. The therapist tone is warm and matter-of-fact. The therapist's is accepting and only slightly questioning of the patient's experience.

Orchestrating an Intense Scene Concerning the Seriousness of the Illness and the Difficulty of Recovery

THERAPIST: So part of you can see that distinction. Now, I want to come back to what it's been like for all of you. You've all described differently just how painful this illness has been for you. You've been panicky, you've been worried, and trying to figure out how to best take care of Susan. Susan has felt preoccupied and out of touch. Both Paul and Dan have described very clearly that they are worried about Susan and about the whole family. And about the amount of energy that has been taken up by all of this. I want to repeat all that because I want to push forward a little bit to giving you a really hard task as parents first. I want you to think very carefully about what you say. Really, you really need to help figure out a way to get Susan over this. She can come back to the hospital, be fed again, and go back out. She can keep doing that over and over again. That happens with some patients. But if you really want to stop it, you're really going to have to figure out a way to get her back to a basic, good nutritional state. And when she's back at that nutritional state, some of the issues that may be underlying this can be explored. If she's healthy enough physically that you can actually get her back into adolescence, where she can actually do things again, think about politics, or friends, or doing things outside of the family without everybody worrying about what she's doing, or if she's safe. Except in the usual teenage way. But right now, you can't do that. You're getting sick with this worry all the time. Now, I'm not expecting Susan to like what I'm saying at all. I hope Susan does, I know the eating disorder won't like what I'm saying. Do you hear the difference?

SUSAN: Yeah.

MOTHER: The Alien.

THERAPIST: Is that what you call it?

SUSAN: That's what my mom refers to it as.

THERAPIST: That's a nice metaphor. You mean in that Sigourney Weaver kind of way? It is kind of an anorectic-looking thing. It's actually a nice metaphor if you think about the kind of strategies and incredible skill it will require to figure out how to deal with this very slippery kind of creature. Now remember, this is not Susan.

MOTHER: No, we know where Susan is. We know when we talk to Susan. And sometimes we don't talk to Susan, sometimes we talk to the Alien. We try to tell Susan through the Alien.

THERAPIST: Sometimes Susan knows?

MOTHER: No, she probably doesn't. Well, I think Susan knows it, but I also think the Alien is pretty stern.

THERAPIST: What do you think about that? Any comment?

SUSAN: No.

THERAPIST: (to Paul and Dan) What about you two?
(No comment, giggling)

FATHER: It's funny because the day Susan went in to the hospital, they indicated to us that they were taking her in to remove the Alien.

DAN: I did?

MOTHER: You did.

FATHER: Dan didn't think it was funny, but I always pretend to take them in to the hospital to get the aliens out, it's a plot.

PAUL: I didn't even know I said that.

FATHER: He was kind of prophetic in what he was saying, though he didn't understand what was going on.

THERAPIST: How did the hospital take the Alien out?

SUSAN: I was fattened, I was fattened up.

THERAPIST: What the hospital can do is take you away from death's door. But the Alien still is there, in the sense that we're talking about. I want you to imagine for a minute that Susan had a cancer that had a 15% mortality rate. What would you do? As parents what would you do?

MOTHER: Actually it's probably easier to deal with because there's things that you can do, and some things you can't. I mean obviously you would seek treatment, you would . . . the cancer. You would do the chemotherapy, you would do all those things that you needed to do, and you would pray.

Charging the Parents with the Task of Refeeding

THERAPIST: And you can do all those things with this illness, too.

MOTHER: I don't think she'd let me . . . I might try.

THERAPIST: As far as I know there is not a cancer involved, but you are seeking treatment, you are making a big effort to be here, I know it. And that's a really good sign as a family, in my opinion. And the dedication that it takes to come here and do those things, not just here in particular, but here this clinic too. That's one thing. But, also there are things you can do as parents. You used to know how to feed her when she was sick, I think you can still figure out some things.

MOTHER: The nasogastric tube comes to mind

THERAPIST: That comes to mind? What is that? You mean am I recommending it? No. But I'm saying, you actually have unique skills to bring because you're her mother. And you 're in business, you might know something about order and discipline, you know, you might need these things. This is not about Susan, this is about anorexia. And until she gets to a reasonable weight and is eating without difficulty, and you can trust her, you are going to have to be on her, in some way. On her in the sense of fighting the anorexia. Now I'm not going to give you a prescription of how to do that. You're her parents, you know her. And you're responsible for her in a sense. And you love her as no one else does.

The therapist makes clear to the parents what their task it but will not tell them specifically how they ought to refeed their daughter. It is important to bring the parents to the task but to allow them to work out for themselves, given the circumstances at home, how best to succeed in this difficult task.

SUSAN: I don't think that punishing me by not letting me go to the mall is a good solution.

THERAPIST: I haven't heard that as a proposal. Is that one that you think is possible?

SUSAN: Well, that's what she said when she heard that I was unstable in clinic.

MOTHER: I said that you could not go to the mall because you were unstable and needed to conserve your calories. And therefore you did not need to be exercising by running all over the mall.

SUSAN: Running all over the mall (*laughing*).

MOTHER: Hey, whatever, it takes energy.

THERAPIST: So one of the things I want to reinforce is that the two of you need to be on the same page (*addressing the parents as a couple*). On the exact same line on a page. About everything you do. Because any slipup gives anorexia nervosa more of a chance at taking over Susan's life and will make it not work. I also want your brothers to help you, Susan. It sounds to me, Susan, that you have amazing brothers.

While reinforcing the parental authority here, the therapist also turns to the siblings for help. Their task is to be supportive of their sister in this ordeal, not to help their parents in the task of refeeding, but to provide their sister with comfort and understanding. This is done also with the aim of extricating the patient from the parental subsystem and realigning her with the sibling subsystem, which becomes more of a theme in subsequent sessions, though the groundwork can be laid here.

SUSAN: I do, if only they would shower regularly, they would be all right.

THERAPIST: They love you very much it seems.

FATHER: They absolutely worship her.

PAUL: Well not worship. . . .

FATHER: In a metaphorical sense. The sun sets and rises on their sister.

THERAPIST: Maybe they know some ways to support Susan and can be supportive to you through their relationship as brothers. Can you think about that? What can you do to help Susan? What are some things you could do?

PAUL: He can wash his hair.

THERAPIST: Well, maybe if that would make her feel better. Do you like his hair to be clean?

MOTHER: He can wash his hair if you'll drink. . . .

SUSAN: That's okay, it's not exactly like equal swap.

MOTHER: Sure it is. It's just as important that he washes his hair as it is to him . . . to him that you eat.

SUSAN: It's not that important to me. I don't have to see him, you know.

THERAPIST: Well, maybe that's not a good example but there are things that they could do. Either of them. Spending time with you, for example. When it's difficult. Doing things with you. Do you like to do things with them?

SUSAN: (*nodding*)

PAUL: Depends on what things.

THERAPIST: Non–anorexia nervosa, laxative abusive, purging kinds of things. Susan things. The things that you, the special commonality between the three of you, reinforces being helpful because these two are going to be working together against anorexia nervosa, and all three of you can help, too.

SUSAN: I think I'm being forced into this. . . .

THERAPIST: Well, maybe. If it was easy, if you could just go *clap* and make anorexia go away, you probably would. Right? I know that, I think your parents and brothers know, too. But they want to help you fight it. Will you let them? Sometimes?

SUSAN: I guess. I don't want to be sick for the rest of my life. I don't want to be sick at all.

Toward the end of this maneuver, the therapist tries to confront the patient's resistance to the proposed treatment. In so doing, he tries to respect the reality of her experience while at the same time suggesting that she, too, has some wish for change.

Preparing for the Next Session's Family Meal and Ending the Session

THERAPIST: I want to show you a lifetime curve (*drawing an imaginary curve in the air*). Here's at age 15, and here's age 30, and people who develop anorexia nervosa have about 3 years before there's just hardly any recovery after that point. So it's important to work on it now . . . all of you, and really dedicate your resources to it. And you may have to take some time away from things you ordinarily would do. But in the long run it's going to save time, and it's going to save Susan. Think about those things. Let me tell you what I want you to do for next time. Next time I want you to bring a picnic, I want you to bring something for everybody to eat and what you believe Susan needs to eat. What you want her to eat, to get well. The idea is, you're in charge of trying to help her get better because she's not able to do it on her own. She's told us that it's a tough battle. She's fighting quite a bit of it, too, but she needs your help. So what we'll do is, we'll come in here, and we'll have a picnic. I won't be eating, so you don't have to bring things for me. But you will all be eating, and I will talk to you during the process about that. Next Friday.

All right, let me summarize the session today. One thing is, I've gotten some sense, a little from each of you, about the warmth and care for one another in your family. The second is that it sounds like everyone is worried, in various ways. All the way from fear to panic to concern about really life and death issues which are facing the family. And then we talked about separating Susan from the illness. We can be clear that it's really the illness we're working against. And we want Susan to recover and get back to her life. And third, we talked about the need for the two of you (*to the parents*) to really examine carefully over this next week how you can work together to ensure that Susan gets the help she needs, to do whatever it takes for a period of time to make sure this happens. Okay, thank you. I appreciate you coming, and I'll see you next week with your picnic.

The therapist ends the session with a good summary of the therapeutic tasks he had to cover in the first session: (1) getting to know each member of the family; (2) emphasizing the seriousness of the illness and reinforcing their concern; (3) separating the illness from the patient; and (4) letting the parents know about the serious task of refeeding they have to embark upon.

6

Session 2: The Family Meal

*S*ession 2 involves a family meal. At the end of Session 1, the parents were instructed to bring in a meal for their daughter that they felt met the nutritional requirements to help with her starved state. In Session 2, the therapist hopes to build on their understanding of the patient and family, as well as provide hope that the family can succeed in refeeding their daughter. The assessment of the family is not a single occurrence; rather, further understanding comes throughout treatment. With the family meal, though, the therapist wants to start his or her assessment of the family's transactional patterns during eating and to help persuade the parents to have their daughter eat one bite more than she is prepared to, while making sure the patient feels supported by her siblings through this ordeal.

The major goals for this session are:

- To continue the assessment of the family structure and its likely impact on the ability of the parents to successfully refeed their daughter.
- To provide an opportunity for the parents to experience success in refeeding their daughter.
- To assess the family process specifically during eating.

In order to accomplish these goals, the therapist undertakes the following interventions during this session:

1. Weighing the patient.
2. Taking a history and observing the family patterns during food preparation, food serving, and family discussions about eating, especially as it relates to the patient.
3. Helping the parents convince their daughter to eat at least one mouthful more than she is prepared to, or helping to set the parents on their way to working out between themselves how they can best go about refeeding their daughter.
4. Aligning the patient with her siblings for support.
5. Closing the session.

Weighing the Patient

The session begins, as all sessions in the first two phases do, with the patient being weighed by the therapist. A report of this weight to the family helps set the tone of the session. If the patient is doing well, then the tone will be more optimistic, whereas if there is a decline in weight or lack of progress, the tone may well be more foreboding.

Taking a History and Observing the Family Patterns during Food Preparation, Food Serving, and Family Discussions about Eating, Especially as It Relates to the Patient

Why

The assessment of the family is obviously not a single occurrence; instead, it is an ongoing process that brings an enriched understanding as treatment progresses. Generalizations of interaction patterns (e.g., cross-generational problems, poor parental alliances, importance of separation of identity) in families are often confusing. For instance, attempts to make Minuchin's (Minuchin et al., 1975) descriptions of psychosomatic families operational to produce measurements have largely been unsuccessful (Dare et al., 1990; Dare, Le Grange, Eisler, & Rutherford, 1994). The importance of these generalizations, though, is that they are often the targets of family therapy. The therapeutic meal offers the therapist an opportunity to observe in vivo these family processes specifically as they are brought to the fore during a meal. The observations gleaned from this family meal help the therapist to identify and plan strategies to intervene with unhealthy interaction patterns that contribute to the maintenance of pathological eating behaviors. Ultimately, during the succeeding sessions, the therapist wants to disrupt unproductive alliances, for example, between the patient and a parent, in order to get the parents to act together in a compelling fashion. Such cross-generational alliances occur when one parent takes a firm, insistent stance on compelling the patient to eat, whereas the other parent becomes an ally of the patient's symptoms, arguing that the quantities of food are too great or the caloric content of a meal is too high. Forming these alliances rather than interparental ones is counterproductive.

Knowledge of the family structure, that is, the often-repeated patterns of communicating, controlling, nurturing, socializing, forming boundaries, making alliances and coalitions, and solving problems, is gained throughout the family meetings but may become more obvious during the family meal. The family meal provides strong exposure to the family's characteristic organization. Similarly, an understanding of the significance of the family patterns and the patient's symptoms should aid the therapist's effectiveness in producing family changes. Symptoms are not believed to be the result of a specific family structure. However, there may be patterns of family interaction that render a family powerless in the presence of symptoms. A patient with an eating disorder cannot improve unless and until there is a change in dietary patterns. In other words, anorexic patients must gain weight to get better. Family therapy is effective not because it undoes a hypothetical family etiology but rather because it changes the way a family responds and manages their daughter's eating disorder.

With adolescent patients, the aim is to set up a meal regimen similar to that in a well-functioning inpatient treatment setting for eating disorders. The parents must be coached to set up a culture such that eating and completing a meal occurs within a set period of time, while the expectation for that occurrence is relentless and powerful. In other words, there is no alternative for the patient other than to comply with her parents' wishes.

How

First, the family is instructed to proceed in laying out the picnic lunch. The therapist does not participate in the meal; instead, he or she takes part in learning more about the family's style during eating by observing the family ritual and by asking questions about eating. For example, the therapist may ask the parent who is serving the food whether that is typical of the pattern at home, whether the food they brought represents the kind of meal they would have had as a family lunch in their dining room, who prepares the food at home, who does the food shopping, and so forth. The reason for this inquiry is to help the therapist and family understand what potential changes in these activities would be advisable.

The therapist should constantly encourage the discovery of new patterns of family interactions by direct instructions and by the way in which he or she addresses the family and constructs the family meetings. For instance, the therapist may prevent family members from speaking for one another or saying that they know what another family member is thinking or feeling. Instead, the therapist should provide an opportunity for each family member to speak for him- or herself or question another as to how they may know what the other is thinking. The therapist, above all, has been observing the process of family interactions and now has an opportunity to observe directly how the family interacts during eating in general and concerning the eating disorder in particular. The therapist has made several appraisals, assessing the mental state of the patient and the characteristics of all the family members while meeting with the family during the preceding sessions.

Helping Parents Convince Their Daughter to Eat at Least One Mouthful More than She Is Prepared to, *or* Helping to Set Parents on Their Way to Working Out How They Can Best Go about Refeeding Their Daughter

Why

One aim of the family picnic is for the therapist to help the parents make their daughter eat at least one mouthful more than she is prepared to. This symbolic act is important, and the family meal may have to last as long as it takes to achieve this goal. The therapist seldom has to achieve more with the family meal, as the effect is striking and the patient now knows that her parents have a new resource in refeeding her.

Thereafter, the parents feel more empowered with the knowledge that they may find it easier to get their daughter to eat more, and, although the struggle may continue for several more months, parental power to enforce more food intake alters the relationship among the patient, parents, and food. The therapist hopes to enforce change by disrupting old and familiar patterns, taking advantage of the family's disorientation in the strange setting of family therapy and under the impact of the therapeutic bind.

Helping the patient eat first before exploring the patient's attitudes and beliefs and her relationship with her family may seem like putting the cart before the horse. However, the therapist needs to point out that, although the latter approach may seem to be the kindest and the one that minimizes conflict, it does not happen with the reliability and predictability that would assure the rescue of their daughter's health. Instead, the therapist should consistently suggest to the parents what they might have to do to get their daughter to eat more than she ordinarily would have. In doing so, he or she reinforces joint parental action, aligns the parents with one another, and begins to remove the patient from the parental subsystem. The authoritative style of the therapist helps the parents to follow his or her guidance. The parents' success in feeding their daughter marks an important turning point for the family; the parents feel empowered that they have managed to begin to defeat the eating disorder and feel invigorated to continue with this task, whereas the patient may experience a sense of relief that her parents have shown the stamina to overcome the demands of the eating disorder. The patient's attitudes and beliefs about eating, as well as her relationship with her family, are indirectly explored throughout Phase I of treatment. The patient's relationship with her family will receive more direct attention in Phase II of treatment, once consistent weight gain has been established. Finally, it is important to point out that the refeeding process primarily belongs to the parents; that is, the therapist should direct comments about this area primarily to the parents. Siblings play a different role in this process, one that we will describe at a later point.

How

The family picnic is an extremely varied occasion, as each family displays its own feeding and mealtime rituals. Many families bring a frugal special meal for their anorexic offspring that is not in keeping with her severe state of starvation while catering appropriately for themselves. At this point, the therapist may remind the family, "You have to provide your daughter, who is starving, with the kinds of food that would restore her weight to normal. Giving her this amount, or this kind of food [in reference to the portions they brought for their daughter], will not correct the starvation." The therapist has to help the parents delve into their knowledge about appropriate feeding of a growing child and can say, "It is full cream milk and pasta with a cream sauce that will make the difference, not a salad."

At the same time, the therapist instructs the parents to take charge of their starving offspring's eating by giving her an amount of food that could begin to reverse the starvation. The avoidance of confrontation and conflict that characterizes the family's customary approach to dieting behavior is usually apparent at the outset. The therapist suggests that the parents sit on either side of the patient and advises them not to discuss the type or amount of food to be eaten but to take action by filling the daughter's plate. The therapist consistently coaches the parents by making repetitive and insistent suggestions as to how to act uniformly, so as to compel the parents to increase gradually the monotonous force applied to their daughter to get her to eat. While "coaching" the parents, it is sometimes necessary and useful for the therapist to physically stand behind the parents and provide them with specific suggestions, much like a prompter. It is often helpful to remind the parents of a time when their daughter was even younger and ill in bed with a bad head cold and the parents tried to get her to eat or to take her medicine. The therapist may say, "You would have found a way to get her to eat," or "You know how to feed a starving child and you don't need expert nutritional advice" in an attempt to bolster their confidence in this task. This procedure is sometimes inelegant, humiliating, and inappropriate given their daughter's age, but getting her to eat that one mouthful more than she was prepared to often marks a turning point.

Aligning the Patient with Her Siblings for Support

Why

Cross-generational instead of interparental alliances are often observed in families with an anorexic youngster. The role of the therapist is to allow the parents to work out a way to operate together as a team (interparental alliance) in order to refeed their adolescent offspring. The therapist should oppose unhealthy family structures, especially those that confuse communication, disrupt powerful parental control, obscure clear cross-generational boundaries, and/or interfere with the maintenance of clear separateness of identity (Dare & Eisler, 1992). For instance, one parent may take on a firm, insistent role in compelling the patient to eat, whereas the other parent becomes an ally to the patient's symptoms, arguing that it is not possible for her to eat that much. This type of cross-generational alliance, instead of an interparental one, should be opposed and/or confronted.

While the parents are being empowered, the role assigned to siblings is one that does not interfere with the parents and their task at hand. Instead, the siblings are reinforced for uncritical support and sympathy for the patient, that is, for establishing healthy cross-generational boundaries in aligning the patient with her siblings as opposed to being coopted into a parental alliance that will ultimately sustain the eating disorder.

The reasons the therapist wants to assign the patient to her sibling subsystem are clearly described in the work of Minuchin et al. (1975). The patient cannot overcome her eating disorder unless the therapist can succeed in extricating her from her coopted position in the parental subsystem and "demote" her to her sibling subsystem. In single-child families, the therapist follows the same principle but may have to emphasize that the patient should find a friend or cousin whom she can confide in. The therapist's aim is clear; he or she wants to get the parents to work together and reinforce healthy intergenerational boundaries between the parental subsystem and the sibling subsystem and also to support the adolescent's development of an appropriate support system.

How

The therapist must both support the joint parental efforts to refeed their daughter and demonstrate his or her understanding of the patient's dreadful predicament—being consumed by her eating disorder, having the therapist "unleash" her parents to take away her only sense of identity and power, and feeling entirely unsupported while this is going on around her. The therapist will say to the patient (and indirectly address her siblings), "While Mom and Dad make every effort to fight your illness and nourish you back to health, you will think that they are being awful to you. You will need to be able to tell someone just how bad things are for you, that is, you will need someone like your brother or sister or school friend who could listen to your complaints." Likewise, the therapist will turn to the patient's siblings and encourage them to be supportive of their sister, not in her efforts to be anorexic but in comforting her when she feels overwhelmed by the turn of events.

Closing the Session

The session should be ended on an optimistic note, congratulating the parents and the family on their efforts, almost regardless of their actual material success. The parents must experience the session as giving them more hope and encouragement about what they can do to help their child. Most sessions should end with a positive note, though when there has been slippage or failure to gain needed weight, more cautionary reminders may also be made in order to keep the family vigilant about the seriousness of not following through on their refeeding initiatives.

End-of-Session Review

The lead therapist should communicate his or her findings and expectations from this meeting to the other team members. In addition, he or she should review with the treatment and consultation team the following questions.

Common Questions for Session 2

What if the family fails to bring a picnic lunch?

This happens very infrequently, but when it does, the therapist should express his or her concern that this failure may delay the family's action in starting the refeeding process. The therapist should explore, in a noncritical manner, what prevented them from taking this important step. The therapist may have to spend the session reinvigorating the parents to take on this awesome task.

What if the family provides themselves with healthy portions of food while serving a meager portion to their anorexic daughter?

The therapist uses this opportunity to guide the parents to reassess the caloric value of the portions they want their starving daughter to eat and aims to get them to realize that unhealthy or meager portions are not sufficient to bring about a steady rise in their anorexic daughter's weight and an eventual restoration of her health. The therapist assists the parents through his or her persistent guidance, and in spite of the patient's protestations, to decide together how much a starving person should be eating in order to regain weight. In some cases, a therapist might suggest actually bringing two meals—one that reflects what the parents believe their daughter should eat and another that reflects what they believe she will eat. This can help to concretely illustrate the discrepancy between where they are starting and what they need to achieve in the refeeding process.

What if the therapist becomes emotionally involved with the family?

Making an assessment of the family often depends on the way in which the therapist becomes absorbed into the family. This sometimes happens because our social training often leads us to accommodate ourselves to the family pattern. This allows us to adjust our role and style to fit in with that of the family. Because the risk of unconsciously fitting into the family patterns that may render the family ineffective in overcoming the patient's eating disorder is professionally potentially hazardous, a cotherapist, supervising peer, or observing team is important. The role of the supervisor is to modify and develop the therapist's direct response to the patient's family.

What if the parents do not succeed in getting their daughter to eat that one mouthful more than she was prepared to?

The therapist uses this opportunity to reinvigorate the parents to take prompt and persistent action to encourage their daughter to eat once they return home (e.g., make similar efforts to feed their daughter when they sit down for their next meal; see Session 3 prescriptions). The therapist also uses this event to demonstrate to the parents once more how powerful the illness is and what drastic efforts are required to rescue their daughter. The therapist should urge the parents not to feel despondent and to try to follow his or her guidelines about refeeding in the next few days. It is essential for the therapist to bolster the parents' skills at feeding their starving child, and she or he may say, "You have done an excellent job until the illness has outsmarted everyone, and because you are successful with your other children in this regard, there is no reason why you should not also be able to regain your efficiency in refeeding your starving daughter."

What if the patient becomes too ill to be treated outside the hospital?

If the therapist experiences difficulty in getting the parents to refeed their starving daughter and restore her weight, the patient may become too ill to be treated outside the hospital. The therapist has to use his or her best judgment here to determine at what juncture he or she recommends that the patient should be hospitalized. This, of course, is an unfortunate turn of events and may complicate treatment on several levels. First, obtaining a bed in a special eating-disorders inpatient unit may prove quite a challenge. Second, the parents may experience a move to an inpatient facility as a further failure on their part, and the patient may become more entrenched in her eating disorder. Third, once the patient is discharged from the hospital, reengaging the family in an effort to mobilize them to make another attempt at this difficult task may prove unsuccessful. Clearly, the therapist should work hard to prevent this scenario from unfolding. However, from time to time it may happen that the therapist has to make arrangements for inpatient treatment. The criteria for inpatient treatment given in Chapter 2 may be two helpful.

After a patient is hospitalized, it is still possible to continue the family therapy approach used in this manual. For example, the occasion of the hospitalization may be additional evidence that the eating problem is severe and that requires the parents to devote themselves to the effort of overcoming the disorder. It can serve as a new crisis to encourage aggressive action. On the other hand, a hospital admission may be experienced as a failure on the part of the family and the therapist. Such a perspective is not helpful and should be avoided. Instead, focus should be maintained on the need for the parents to pick up the refeeding process after their child is discharged.

Because the family is unlikely to be able to participate in the actual refeeding process of a hospitalized child, the emphasis on any family work should be on the seriousness of the medical problems their child is experiencing and the need for action on the parents' part to turn this around. Continuing to support the parents in developing feelings of empowerment may be difficult in a hospital setting, but such support should be undertaken. It is likely that family therapy in the hospital, therefore, must be more limited in scope.

What if the patient eats well during this session?

The patient may undermine the impact of the family meal by eating well. As pointed out previously, the parents should have an experience of success in this session. If the patient eats, we miss the therapeutic opportunity to give the parents a direct experience of empowerment. They may have been defeated by the eating disorder for several years, and this may be their first opportunity to feel that they can control their child's illness. Therefore, it is useful to ask the patient to resist the parents' attempts at getting her to eat during the family meal. The therapist may say, "I realize that you would like to be of help to your parents because it often upsets you that your parents are struggling so much. I am sure that there is a part of you that is very frightened that your eating disorder is so powerful that you can make them unable to stop you from starving yourself, even to death. It must also be humiliating for you to be seen to be made to eat. So, having said all that, I would like for you to try as hard as you can to stop your parents feeding you, because I don't want you to let go of your admirable tenacity or your independent vitality. What I do want, though, is for you to be physically safe and to find healthier ways to use your strength of character and individuality. As I have said, I do not want you to give up fighting for yourself. I think you need to be stronger to fight for yourself. That's why you need to be properly nourished." This intervention has the quality of a paradoxical injunction—that is, if the patient complies, she is doing what the therapist asked her to do, and if she does not comply (if she eats), she does so at the parents' command, which is also what the therapist ultimately wants her to do as well. It should be noted that AN is felt by patients to be a "friend," a supportive, valuable presence. Taking away AN is depriving her of something she values. This can be acknowledged and the patient's point of view accepted as her genuine belief and need.

What if the patient eats more than she planned to early in the session?

It may happen that the patient succumbs relatively early to the pressures the parents are placing on her to eat more than she had planned. If this occurs, although the explicit behavioral goal of the session has been reached, that is, the patient has eaten one more bite than she had planned, there remains an opportunity to educate, support, and encourage the parents in their efforts during this session. In other words, continue to empower and push the parents in learning how to refeed their daughter.

7

Session 2 in Action

*T*his chapter provides an example of Session 2. It begins with a short background on the patient and her family. The session is divided into major parts by the interventions. In addition, as the session unfolds, explanatory text guides the reader as to the aims the therapist has in mind.

To review, the major goals for Session 2 are:

- To continue the assessment of the family structure and its likely impact on the ability of the parents to successfully refeed their daughter.
- To provide an opportunity for the parents to experience success in refeeding their daughter.
- To assess the family process specifically during eating.

In order to accomplish these goals, the therapist undertakes the following interventions during this session:

1. Weighing the patient.
2. Taking a history and observing the family patterns during food preparation, food serving, and family discussions about eating, especially as it relates to the patient.
3. Helping parents convince their daughter to eat at least one mouthful more than she is prepared to, or helping to set par-

ents on their way to working out how they can best go about refeeding their daughter.
4. Aligning the patient with her siblings for support.
5. Closing the session.

Clinical Background

Rhonda is the 17-year-old only child of an intact family. She was diagnosed with AN approximately 4 months prior to beginning family therapy. She required hospitalization for severe malnutrition and medical instability for approximately 4 weeks. In the past, Rhonda also occasionally binged and purged, though these events are rare at this point. Neither of Rhonda's parents was married previously, and they have no other children. They both work in the local area and do not travel for business. Rhonda is a good student and works hard to succeed in school. She reports that her eating disorder began after peers noted that she had lost weight and complimented her on her looks.

Weighing the Patient

The session begins with the patient being weighed. It is noted that her weight has decreased from the previous session. The therapist uses this opportunity to check with the adolescent about how she feels about her progress this past week and to assess her reaction to weight gain or loss. This helps the therapist to gauge something of the patient's reaction to the parents' refeeding efforts and also serves as an opportunity for the therapist to cultivate a relationship with the patient.

The family has brought a picnic meal with them and begins to take it out of the containers.

Taking a History and Observing the Family Patterns during Food Preparation, Food Serving, and Family Discussions about Eating Especially as It Relates to the Patient

MOTHER: So, we're supposed to eat?

THERAPIST: Yes.

FATHER: And what else? Aren't you going to ask us any questions?

THERAPIST: Yes. We'll talk while you're eating.

FATHER: Okay, great. We had no idea what to bring because there was no microwave or anything, so we went over to the deli.

THERAPIST: Who all went to the deli?

FATHER: My wife and I.

MOTHER: But we took down orders. We took down orders.

FATHER: Yeah, last night.

THERAPIST: So you talked about it last night?

MOTHER: Oh, yeah. So that's what I tried to get.

THERAPIST: Can you tell me how it has been going this week?

FATHER: We went to the hotel on Sunday for a champagne brunch. I haven't seen Rhonda eat that much food in a long time. She did great. She had everything from salads to really rich chocolate desserts. She did really good, really good.

MOTHER: And she saw X [celebrity] there with his wife. He came by the hospital when she was hospitalized.

RHONDA: He went around 'cause his leg was broken, so he went around with his wife. His wife is beautiful. I recognized his wife, and I went up to her and I said "Hi," and then I went up to him and I said, "Hi." They didn't really remember me 'cause of my haircut, but then they go, "Ohh."

THERAPIST: Exciting.

RHONDA: She's very nice.

THERAPIST: You felt very lucky. Huh?

RHONDA: And Y [another celebrity] came, too.

THERAPIST: All on separate days?

RHONDA: They signed hats and stuff.

THERAPIST: Was this at Christmas?

RHONDA: Or, was it after? Maybe it was after.

THERAPIST: Do you often eat out, or do you mostly eat at home?

FATHER: Mostly at home. We eat out mainly on the weekend.

MOTHER: When we have more time.

FATHER: 'Cause we enjoy going out to breakfast and dinner on the weekends, have somebody serve us.

FATHER: Especially breakfast.

As the family goes about serving themselves, the therapist engages them in conversation about eating and makes an assessment of their eating both here in the office and in their family home and elsewhere. The therapist is trying initially to encourage general conversation (football, celebrities, etc.) in order to help the family relax a little. The situation of eating in front of others can feel quite awkward. At the same time, the therapist want things to proceed as normally as possible, so the therapist is not as active in the early part of the session as he becomes later on once some information has come out.

MOTHER: No onions [*referring to the sandwich*]. We went to the deli, I saw chicken salad, potato salad. I said, uh-oh, what are we going to do? Because I didn't see tuna salad. So I asked the lady, and she says, "Oh yeah, we have tuna salad."

THERAPIST: (*to Rhonda*) Do you have a tuna salad sandwich?

RHONDA: Yeah. I've been eating fish lately.

FATHER: This is kind of funny, eating in front of other people watching. Usually when you eat, people are eating with you.

THERAPIST: My job is to do something different, it's to talk to you about it.

FATHER: It doesn't bother me.

THERAPIST: So normally at home . . . I noticed that you (*to mother*) took things out of the bag and handed them out. Do you serve at home?

RHONDA: Umm. Sometimes mainly my dad serves.

THERAPIST: Is that the tradition in your house?

FATHER: I don't know, maybe because I do the cooking, or most of the cooking.

THERAPIST: There you go.

FATHER: That could be, or Rhonda. She doesn't cook [*referring to mother*].

MOTHER: I can cook, but I just don't do it well.

THERAPIST: So this was sort of typical in that sense. You didn't cook it but you sort of dished it out. This is the role that you've come to have. Has it always been that way since Rhonda was born, that you (*to father*) mostly cook?

RHONDA: My mom makes grilled cheese sandwiches.

FATHER: No, she used to cook more, but now she doesn't.

MOTHER: I guess just never finding the time. Because I'm so tired when I come home from work, because I work in the city, and by the time I come home it's late.

RHONDA: She does come home an hour and a half after my dad.

FATHER: (*to his mother*) And you're more stressed than me.

MOTHER: I don't take it out on anyone at work. I just say, "I had a lousy day, as usual." That's fine. "Okay, what about you and tell me about work and how was your school." I concentrate on them, I don't bring my problems home.

RHONDA: It's usually I bring all my school problems home.

THERAPIST: (*to Rhonda*) You talk to them about them?

RHONDA: Just, like, at the dinner table or something. If I have problems with a teacher. Which I didn't really, except just one teacher out of my 4 years. That was last year. I'm usually the one talking about school and stuff like that.

THERAPIST: So, what's a typical meal, Rhonda, that you would have? You guys share it, right?

RHONDA: Actually, lately I haven't really been having what they've been having. Because when they have meat or something like that. I haven't really been having meat. After I got out of the hospital, I have, like, beans. Because beans are really high in protein, Power Bars, and Boost. Mainly for protein. I don't like a lot of meat. Well, I do like meat. It's just that I haven't been eating it, I've been having, like, vegetarian burgers and stuff like that. Just not a lot of meat.

MOTHER: You got the idea of vegetarian burgers from the hospital.

RHONDA: Uh-huh, because that was the first time I'd had them, was in the hospital, and I liked that.

THERAPIST: Are those garden burgers?

RHONDA: Yeah, I get garden burgers, and the ones in the hospital are vegetarian burgers.

MOTHER: It's the same concept.

THERAPIST: So when you cook a meal, what kinds of things do you cook?

RHONDA: That I'll eat or that I just cook for, like . . . ?

THERAPIST: Well, that's interesting, you cook things that you don't eat?

RHONDA: Yeah.

THERAPIST: What would you cook first, then we'll talk about what you'll eat.

RHONDA: I like to cook, as far as ethnic foods, I like to cook American, Italian, and Asian.

FATHER: She's a good cook, real good.

THERAPIST: Are there particular dishes that you tend to make more than others?

RHONDA: As far as for meals, no.

THERAPIST: Favorite recipes?

RHONDA: I like making bread from scratch, and pastries, 'cause I like, I love fixing stuff fancy. For Thanksgiving, I made pumpkin pie, and I fixed a nice tray of cookies. I like to arrange things, and put garnish just to make the plate look pretty.

THERAPIST: So when you serve the dinners that you make, do you serve it on a plate, you plate the food and serve it like a restaurant?

RHONDA: Uh-huh. I love doing that.

FATHER: She won't let us into the kitchen when she cooks. We have to be sitting at the table. And she'll dish everybody's food out.

THERAPIST: Just like a restaurant.

RHONDA: I don't like, even though we have a pretty good size kitchen, it feels crowded when someone's in there trying to do something while I'm cooking. So I'm like, I don't want anyone in here.

THERAPIST: (*to father*) How about you, what kinds of things do you usually cook?

FATHER: Anything.

THERAPIST: Do you have a specialty?

FATHER: No, not really, chicken, London broil, steak.

THERAPIST: Do you serve it on the plates too or do you put it in a dish and serve it family style?

FATHER: Most of the time I'll serve it. Since Rhonda came home from the hospital, I don't serve Rhonda. We'll just let her, she picks what she wants to eat, she'll fix it herself, or in the kitchen, then she takes it to the table.

This information is helpful for the therapist in seeing how the family has accommodated themselves to "make room" for the eating disorder. Note that the therapist makes an attempt to "interview" all of the members of the family during this process, looking for differences of opinion, as well as points of reference that may suggest strategies that will help the family in the refeeding process ahead. In this case, the therapist notes particularly the heightened role of the father both in the preparation and serving of the food. This may help the family when they are actively encouraging their daughter to eat. The therapist also notes that Rhonda is cooking "for others" and that this pattern will likely need to be changed. The therapist tries to take full advantage of the disorientation that the "odd situation" of eating in a clinical setting provides.

MOTHER: But if she does eat what we're eating, or some of the stuff, we'll ask her how much she wants, and she tells us.

FATHER: Or she dishes it out herself.

RHONDA: I like potatoes, I like potatoes a lot.

FATHER: How is it [*referring to the sandwich*]?

RHONDA: It's good.

MOTHER: How is your sandwich on the Dutch Crunch?

FATHER: It's good.

MOTHER: It's not as messy. . . .

FATHER: I'm hungry.

RHONDA: My grandma is out there, she is eating by herself. It's funny, she's like sitting in the corner. Last time the guard came up to her because they thought something was wrong.

THERAPIST: Does she normally live at your house?

FATHER: No, she lives in Cincinnati.

THERAPIST: Oh, she's visiting. So, it wouldn't be typical for her to be eating with you. This is more typical. The three of you.

RHONDA: She actually was supposed to come out, when I was admitted in to the hospital, and then. . . .

THERAPIST: (*to mother*) This is your mom?

MOTHER: This is my mom, yeah.

RHONDA: Actually my other grandparents, my dad's parents, they live five minutes away from us. But we don't really see them so much. I'll go over there sometimes, and maybe have coffee and play cards and stuff, but we don't, like, eat, except on special occasions. We more or less just visit, not formal or anything.

It is vital to establish whether any other member or members of the extended family play an important part in the family's mealtimes. In this instance, the therapist tries to understand what role the respective grandparents may fulfill in everyday eating in this family. The therapist determines that, although the grandmother is currently in the house, she is not a usual member and that the family has made the right decision in not including her in this session.

THERAPIST: Do you ever have people over, do you socialize?

FATHER: Not a lot, no.

THERAPIST: You're not entertainers?

FATHER: No.

MOTHER: Sometimes we have Rhonda's friends over, occasionally. Like your friend Laura was the last one. Last week I think it was, wasn't it?

RHONDA: Probably, probably last week. I usually don't, I usually don't have, like, my friends over because I like to kind of, if I go out and do something, I like to be out of the house. Like during the summer, I would go to their house every weekend. Since it was summer, I didn't have any summer school or anything. I was there, not every day, but a lot.

THERAPIST: Did you eat at her house?

RHONDA: Like at her house they don't have any certain times that they all eat, they all kind of eat when they want to. So it's kind of casual. A lot of her friends, they just stop by. A lot of her friends I knew very well too. So, they could stop by, and they could have a bite to eat. And sometimes her stepdad would cook, because he was a chef at a Chinese restaurant.

FATHER: Oh really? You never told me that.

RHONDA: So, he'd cook. But, I had oriental food a lot over the summer. But I enjoyed that. I had breads and cereals. They bought this huge box thing, because they knew I liked cereal, and it was little boxes, you know cereals, variety.

THERAPIST: Do you have a set time at your house, for meals?

MOTHER: I don't know. Well, we eat together, whether we eat later, depending on our afternoon chores, but we always eat together.

THERAPIST: Dinner.

MOTHER: At dinner time, yeah.

THERAPIST: Do you have any other meals you usually eat together?

FATHER: Breakfast.

MOTHER: Breakfast, before we go to work and school.

THERAPIST: Do you sit down for breakfast?

MOTHER: No, we stand.

FATHER: In the kitchen, we don't have a lot of time.

THERAPIST: But you're also together?

FATHER: Yeah we are.

RHONDA: Well, it depends, though, well, like now, they go to work and I'm sleeping in because I don't go to school right now. So, I'm with my grandma sometimes, I'll usually get up and eat by myself, because she doesn't get up until really late. Not really late, but later, and we go out for lunch or something. But at first, at first when she came out here, I was just out of the hospital for maybe 3 days, about 3 days. And so when she came out it was hard and I got really angry and stuff, because she was doing everything that I . . . I told all of them I was uncomfortable with. She came out and she was doing the exact opposite. I was kind of aggravated and stuff, but now I'm better.

FATHER: She was just trying to get you to eat.

MOTHER: As my mom would say, she acted with tough love. She has these little kind of corny sayings.

THERAPIST: So you knew it wasn't really critical of you, she was just trying to help you. But it was still hard to hear.

FATHER: We did tell her to back off, and stay out of the situation till we knew what direction we were going in. And she did.

THERAPIST: How long do your meals last?

FATHER: About an hour usually.

THERAPIST: You sit down and you talk about your day?

FATHER: Oh, yeah.

MOTHER: Well, we go out to dinner sometimes, we're at a restaurant two hours. We're still eating dinner, and two or three people at different tables leave while we're still sitting there. We make it a real social event, a family event.

FATHER: I don't like to sit, eat, and run, I never do it.

MOTHER: Even if we go to a place like a sandwich shop or another informal place like that, we're there for a couple hours.

FATHER: You see a lot of people sit down, and I call it, they shovel their food in, and they eat so fast and I think to myself, how can they enjoy it? You know. But I don't know what their lifestyle is either, maybe they don't have much time. I always like to take my time and eat.

THERAPIST: So this is something that's a pattern, you make it a social event, or you make the enjoyment of food part of the process.

FATHER: We always did.

THERAPIST: How have Rhonda's decisions about not eating affected this?

MOTHER: Well, the night before she was admitted to the hospital, which I guess was in November, we just had pasta. Was it pasta with vegetables? That's one of our favorite dishes and it's just a, not a huge helping, but a nice generous helping. And we found out that she wasn't eating very much during the day. We told her, "You've got to eat, you've got to eat." And we sat there for over an hour just to make sure she would eat. She ate most of it, but if we didn't keep after her, she wouldn't have eaten at all. It was very frustrating to us, too, because we didn't want her wasting away, so we had to have her eat something. That was her last substantial meal before she was hospitalized. The morning before she was admitted, we went out and she only had half a plain bagel, and then juice or something, and that was it.

THERAPIST: So before that, things must have been not been going too well, either. Had you been just sort of watching her not eat more and more?

FATHER: No, because actually she did eat at the table most of the time when she was sitting with us. It was just before she was hospitalized that she stopped. I'd say within a week.

RHONDA: Actually, like, to tell you what was going on inside me . . . I wasn't eating beforehand, I was at the dinner table, and knowing how we eat, we eat, we talk, we do all that, we socialize. But, it was disrupting that because we were arguing and everything, and I didn't like that. So I was just, like, well, I'm going to start to eat, but that's when I started eating and then I'd purge my food. So because I wasn't happy just sitting there refusing to eat, and then they got mad, and then we just, we went and talked like a family. I just ate so there wouldn't be tension.

The therapist tries to keep the focus on the family's eating in the office. Although Rhonda's information here may seem to be a diversion from the therapist's maneuver to get the parents to begin to consider what she should be eating here and now, the patient provides important insight into her inner world, and the therapist respects the sensitivity of this information.

THERAPIST: So, you ate and then you didn't?

RHONDA: But I got tired, yeah, that was basically that. But then I got tired. I didn't like purging my food, I got tired of that so I just didn't eat during the meal, and if it didn't work out I'd just go. I'd just go upstairs and read. And that would make my parents mad obviously, because I'd get up and I'd leave the dinner table, and I'd go upstairs and they'd get upset with that, but I was tired of eating and then getting rid of the food. Because it felt like work to me.

THERAPIST: This is really a difficult situation that I'm hearing about. You were working very hard to have a meal. You were trying to take care of, cook for each other. You were trying to manage all these feelings inside of you, not wanting to eat then having to get rid of it, and wanting to please your parents, not having them mad at you. There is a very complex set of things that were going on there. How long did that go on?

RHONDA: How long did all of this thinking go on?

THERAPIST: Yeah, that sort of stressful situation.

RHONDA: At the dinner table, for a couple months.

FATHER: It was that long?

RHONDA: Because I didn't. . . . Well, because I also wasn't at home all the time even when school started. I wasn't at home sometimes for dinner. I'd have dinner, or I'd tell them I had dinner or something.

THERAPIST: But you didn't? That was another way to get around it?

RHONDA: I may have had cereal. Because they didn't have, and in a way I went over to my friend's house a lot, because I knew they didn't have structured meal plans. And they didn't eat when they were supposed to so it's kind of like nobody noticed.

FATHER: Didn't Laura. . . .

RHONDA: Well, my friend was always saying to me. . . .

FATHER: Because she's a big eater.

RHONDA: Yeah, my friend, like, you know, she's 82 pounds, and she eats a lot, but she has a really good metabolism. But she's a really good eater, and she noticed that I wasn't eating that much, and she said, "You have to eat more," and she'd give me oriental food, some rice and maybe some meat or something. And I would pick at that. One thing I never did was I never was in public and ate and then purged. I never did that in public, never, never at someone else's house, it was when I was always at home. It's possibly because too I had put on makeup and you know lipstick or whatever and I'd ruin the makeup, and I didn't want to do that. That could have been some of it, too, I just never did it in public.

MOTHER: When we first heard of her purging, every time we finished dinner, after we cleaned up or something. You know, we would always follow her upstairs, you know, at least for a little while after she ate.

FATHER: Or sit on the top of the stairs.

MOTHER: Or sit on the top of the stairs, while she was in the bathroom.

FATHER: And then we told her she couldn't close the bathroom door then after awhile. Don't close the bathroom door. You know we're not going to stand there and watch you but we're going to be sitting near.

RHONDA: But then, after they stopped that, because they did stop that after awhile. . . .

THERAPIST: Did that keep you from purging?

RHONDA: Yeah, except in the morning. In the morning, and I told you about that.

FATHER: When she was rushing me out the door, and I never realized what was going on. She never told me that I was going to be late for work before, and I don't really have to be at work at any specific time, I can get there at 7 or 7:30 or whatever. And I did notice that before she was hospitalized she started saying in the morning, "Dad, you're going to be late, hurry up, you're going to be late." To rush me out of the house. And I never put two and two together, until she told me what she was doing.

THERAPIST: What were you doing, Rhonda?

RHONDA: Well, when my dad would leave. . . . It almost was like every day. Because I liked, I didn't like purging, but I liked the other part. What would happen, when my dad would leave I'd hurry up and I'd go downstairs, I'd hurry up and I'd go downstairs. I'd eat like two sweet rolls, I got a bunch of Halloween candy because I went out and I trick-or-treated on Halloween. I'd eat, you know, those little miniature Snickers and stuff.

MOTHER: In the morning?

RHONDA: I'd eat like two of those, two Milky Ways, I'd eat M&M's, I would eat a lot of food, and two sweet rolls, sometimes I'd eat a donut too. But, I would go and purge it, but one day I couldn't. One day I couldn't. This was a while ago, but I couldn't and I went to school and I felt really guilty, because that day I ate the most out of all days and so, and so I called my dad. I went to the health office and I said I didn't feel good, and I called my dad and I told him that. I mean this is something they all know. I told the doctors all about it. I called and I said, "My stomach doesn't feel good I want to go home." And he said maybe it's 'cause you haven't eaten that much and I said maybe. And so I went home, and I tried again, even though it was maybe 2 hours after the fact. I tried again to purge it, and I couldn't, so then I walked down to Safeway, which was not that far, I walked down there and he wanted, and I knew he wanted, like, I don't know, I made an excuse to go down there, he ran out of whipped cream, and he likes it in his coffee and stuff. And we ran out of cookies. And I went down there and I bought that and I walked back, because I felt guilty, so I thought. . . .

MOTHER: So you walked all the way there and back when you got the cookies and Cool Whip?

THERAPIST: Is that a long way?

RHONDA: Not really

FATHER: Well, to walk it, it could be.

MOTHER: Well, there's an uphill, too.

RHONDA: So that wasn't bad, and I took the long way back, I went like around.

THERAPIST: This was to walk it off?

RHONDA: I know I didn't walk it off because it was a lot, you know, I was thinking 270 calories for one sweet roll, and I had two, and I had a donut, and I had all that candy, I mean because when you're eating really fast you can consume a lot and when you stop it expands, and that's what can make you feel uncomfortable.

MOTHER: You had candy in the morning?

RHONDA: Well, because, because I didn't have it any other time, and when I binged, I only binged on stuff I didn't eat any other time, just to feed my craving and then not have it in my body.

THERAPIST: So why did you go to Safeway?

RHONDA: Well, first of all, it was a destination to walk to. So I can walk, and it was something to do, a destination I could go to.

THERAPIST: So, did you want anything?

RHONDA: No.

FATHER: She got stuff for me. Not for her.

At this point, the family recognizes that the eating disorder has caused Rhonda to deceive them even more than they had earlier believed. Although there is a developing sense of shock and dismay at this realization, neither parent responds with anger or criticism. The therapist takes note of these developments because they suggest that the parents, though naïve about how eating disorders are fully affecting their interactions with their daughter, are trying to find a noncritical approach to the problems she is presenting. This may be a hopeful sign for her recovery, because noncritical families seemed to succeed better overall in refeeding their children than those with more hostile and critical ways of interacting (see Eisler et al., 1997).

THERAPIST: Whipped cream and cookies. Do you usually shop for your parents?

RHONDA: I always went to the store every Saturday with my parents, and I still do.

THERAPIST: So you go shopping together? Usually? This meal was planned a little, you took orders? That's what you said?

FATHER: Last night, my wife wrote everything down.

MOTHER: I put what kind of sandwich my mom wanted, and what kind of sandwich Father and Rhonda and I wanted, and drinks. I wrote it all down to make sure I got it right.

THERAPIST: So, typically, you all go shopping together.

MOTHER: Yes, and Rhonda would help us, she would look at the list and say, "I'll get this, this." She'll bring it back.

THERAPIST: Oh, I see, tag-team shopping.

FATHER: Exactly.

RHONDA: And I got stuff, but I also like doing that because it felt like after breakfast I'd go and at least be moving around some, so it wouldn't be like sitting doing nothing. So, I went and I liked that because I was kind of walking around. And also, being in a grocery store, too, you kind of, it may sound strange, but you kind of, like, see the different kinds of foods.

THERAPIST: It doesn't sound strange to me because I've talked to a lot of people who buy things like whipped cream for someone else, things that they wouldn't eat.

RHONDA: I like cooking for my parents, and I saw them eat it, then maybe I'd pick at it, or I wouldn't eat it. Like, I like fixing really nice desserts, really nice things.

THERAPIST: But you wouldn't eat them?

FATHER: Yeah, and they're forced on us.

MOTHER: It would take us 2 weeks to eat the cake.

RHONDA: Because I like cooking baked things just to see how it would turn out.

The family provides a great deal of information about their habits with regard to eating. What they also demonstrate is the degree to which the eating disorder has become a part of their daughter's everyday behavior, and no one might have noticed that. The therapist uses this time to make a detailed assessment of how this family "arranges" themselves regarding the topic of food and food preparation and consumption. For example, the therapist notes that in this family the father does most of both the cooking and the serving. He may be the main person the therapist needs to engage in the specifics of providing a nourishing diet that helps to defeat the hold AN has on his daughter. The therapist also learns that the patient "cooks for others," a familiar strategy by those affected with AN. The parents are being "fattened up" as the patient starves. These types of observations allow the therapist to identify, for use in future sessions, ways in which the family is likely to interact during the refeeding process and allow him to more quickly assist in solving problems that arise.

MOTHER: One thing we learned in the hospital that I wasn't aware of. When you're consuming food, 25% of your food goes out of your body already. Right away, what you are eating, and then it usually takes a half hour to an hour and then after that there is no more food in your system.

FATHER: I was surprised.

THERAPIST: Well, that's why it's very difficult to purge after too long a period.

RHONDA: And I didn't know this.

THERAPIST: You didn't know.

FATHER: I didn't realize that so much was absorbed in the system almost immediately. Because I always thought it took hours.

THERAPIST: To digest?

FATHER: To digest it, but not through the stomach.

THERAPIST: Most of the nutrients are taken up through the intestinal tract, the stomach is kind of like a holding tank. Digestion takes longer. It's that intestine you've seen pictures of it, that long curly thing. It's like a long hose.

FATHER: So, that's the part where all the nutrients are taken out.

RHONDA: That's the part I didn't really like paying attention to.

MOTHER: So, if you're purging 2 hours after you eat, it could just be bile.

The therapist makes use of every opportunity to educate the parents about the eating disorder, for example, providing them (and the patient) with information about the digestive system. Although this type of information may seem basic, it is clearly helpful for this family to have this type of specific information. In this case, the parents' lack of such information has helped them to "collude" with the illness out of unawareness.

The therapist learns that in this family, the daughter is powerful because she is able to keep much of her behavior out of the awareness of her parents. As she has been an unusually compliant and helpful child, the parents have had little practice in managing opposition from her. This makes it more difficult for parents to act decisively to stop the AN behavior. It is also clear, though, that the parents have a great deal of influence over their daughter and fundamentally little criticism of her. Thus the therapist learns the major problems to be confronted using the strategies of this therapy with this family: (1) the parents lack sufficient information about the illness; (2) the parents have little practice confronting opposition in their daughter; and (3) there is no sibling support or other familial support in the home. On the positive side, the therapist learns that (1) the parents have not been preoccupied with weight and shape concerns, so they can more likely be allies in the struggle against AN; (2) the family is supportive, warm, and noncritical which will help the refeeding process proceed with less friction.

Helping Parents Convince Their Daughter to Eat at Least One Mouthful More Than She Is Prepared to, or Helping to Set Parents on Their Way to Working Out How They Can Best Go about Refeeding Their Daughter

THERAPIST: Let me just ask you (*to parents*), do you think ... I don't know if you're finished yet, I'm not pushing you to finish at all ... do you think that the amount of food that she ordered, you bought, is what she needed? That she needs to eat in order to be healthy? Or to make progress towards that?

MOTHER: She told her father earlier today that she was only going to eat half her sandwich because she was pretty full from what she ate already today. As far as her caloric intake today, I don't know how much she has had so far. That drink has no calories (referring to a bottle of water), and a half a sandwich, I don't know how many calories that would be.

THERAPIST: Tuna sandwich with no mayonnaise?

FATHER: Well, there is mayonnaise in the tuna, but we made it with no extra mayonnaise on the bread. I would have been happy if she would have eaten it, I knew she wouldn't, I knew she wouldn't. I was shocked on Sunday when I saw all the food she ate.

THERAPIST: What happened on Sunday, that you were so comfortable eating?

RHONDA: I was hungry.

THERAPIST: Well, that's good, that's a great reason to eat.

MOTHER: I think you enjoyed it, too.

THERAPIST: Was there something different about it that allowed you to be hungry? A great day of some type?

RHONDA: No, I just think that, I don't know.

THERAPIST: Well, you felt free to eat. That's such a good thing. It's good to have that feeling, and when you have this kind of disorder it's hard to have that feeling.

RHONDA: I was just hungry, I don't know, because I probably, I wasn't eating that great in the hospital, in fact I lost a lot. I just figured that I could afford to eat above average.

THERAPIST: Were you conscious about the fat content in the food you were eating? Did you kind of count the calories?

RHONDA: No, but in a way it was weird because it felt like I was bingeing in some way, because. . . . But actually I was eating a lot of good food, but when I got to the dessert part, that's the part I really wanted, and it felt like I was bingeing.

FATHER: And she went wild, that's what surprised me. Rich, dark chocolate cream puffs.

THERAPIST: What was wild?

FATHER: She had a lot.

RHONDA: I had, had two, they were really good cream puffs. They were like top and bottom pastry, with chocolate in the middle, and I ate two of those, and two slices of, like, I don't know, not chocolate pie, but something.

FATHER: Like cheesecake?

RHONDA: It wasn't cheesecake, I had the crust, the bottom. And I ate two of those.

MOTHER: But we all knew, that even for us, it was going to be our only meal, because we ate at 12, and that's all we ate all day. So the calories that Rhonda consumed that day are probably equal to 4 of 5 days of the calories from previous days.

THERAPIST: How did you feel after you ate?

RHONDA: I felt funny, I surprisingly didn't feel guilty, I really didn't. I didn't count out the calories, but that was just that day.

THERAPIST: That would be making a point that it was a special day for some reason in terms of behavior and your thinking, not that it was a birthday. So how did you feel as parents that day, you had taken her to a place where she really enjoyed eating. It must have felt somewhat good?

FATHER: No, because the night before, she hadn't eaten, and she lost weight on Friday night. So, we saw Dr. X and he said he was going to, if she loses more weight on Tuesday, he may have to admit her. That's what he told her, and we heard this, and I heard it the first time right in the room here. On Saturday night, Saturday all day, she really didn't eat anything, hardly anything, maybe 500 tops calories. I didn't say too much about it, but after supper when I saw she didn't eat anything, and she was upstairs, I said which obviously she heard me, that if she goes back into the hospital again, that I was going to sell the horse, and I mean it, I will. And because one of the deals was, when Rhonda, before she went in to the hospital, she said she was going to turn this whole thing around, just before she was admitted, maybe 2 weeks at the most. And, I told Rhonda, she's always wanted a horse, since she was a baby. And I said, "We'll buy you a horse, and all the equipment that goes with it, we'll board it out, and it's very, very expensive." And I said, "We'll go ahead and we'll do it for you, if you," because she said, "I'll make myself better, I'll eat real good, and everything." And we thought she would, and she did at first, and she got the horse, and she was eating really good, and she was very conscious of it. And I would say, it just went downhill, real fast, real fast. I noticed nothing, she hadn't eaten at all during the day. So then she already got the horse, and we're kind of stuck there, because she's doing the opposite of what she told us she would do, and that is not like Rhonda to do that because she always, when she says she's going to do something she follows through. But, I don't want this to continue, for her health because I realize that it's very serious. When I talk to all the doctors and all the nurses, each time there is deterioration, a little bit more each time, the heart muscles get weaker, then they get stronger, then they get weaker, it's obvious, Rhonda's age, they said at 17, don't worry about it, they're very resilient, they'll come right back. But how many times before there could develop a problem, and that's what scares me. And, I'll do anything for Rhonda, she has a brand new car, she picked the car out herself, we went and we bought it for her. She wanted a horse, we went and we bought it for her, but I will sell the horse if she doesn't help herself and she goes back into the hospital again. Because I mean, like you said last week, some girls may tend to use it as a crutch, go back, they're taken care of for X amount of weeks, but ultimately they are going to be in the same situation when they are released. It will go right back to coming back out, they have to do it themselves.

THERAPIST: I think in the hospital, most of the girls don't feel like it's a crutch, they feel like it's a terrible thing to have to be in the hospital. But you're right, psychologically, that may be so. (to Rhonda) You think so, a little bit?

RHONDA: As far as. . . .

THERAPIST: Because you can't be responsible for a while, everybody's there all the time making sure you're doing it, as much as they can. And it's not perfect, as I know you know, there are ways to cheat in the hospital, and not. . . .

RHONDA: And I won't mention any names, but someone was like saying, like ways she's cheated and ways that other girls had and stuff, it's kind of disturbing. If you cheat, there are always ways, not that they'll find out at first, but I mean in the end you're making it worse on yourself.

MOTHER: Did you ever cheat at the hospital?

RHONDA: No, because I wanted to get out, and it still took me 3 weeks and a day, but that was mostly . . . that was 2 weeks.

THERAPIST: One of the things that helping Rhonda at this point continue to make progress, sounds like over the weekend, it was very distressing for you to watch her not eat on Saturday. You wanted to make sure she knew that you were going to take some action. And did you agree with that action, in terms of trying to get her to eat by selling the horse. . . . ?

MOTHER: Definitely, and then after we talked about it, Rhonda came down and she went and got a Boost, and she started drinking and we were sitting in the kitchen, and she came up to us and she said she was thinking that she really wants to get better and she really wants to make a go at this and try harder because she really wants to keep the horse, and she wants to do well in school, she wants to at least graduate high school and go to a junior college to start. Who told you that you had to have a clean bill of health?

RHONDA: Dr. X.

MOTHER: Yeah, to go to college you had to have a clean bill of health.

RHONDA: Or, you can't have anything that is going to discourage you from being able to concentrate.

THERAPIST: Are there other things that you talked about together to try to help Rhonda? We talked about that last time.

MOTHER: Well, we would always say, if we have a certain dinner, Rhonda can make herself a veggie-burger, so what if she eats something different as long as she has some nutrients and a good balanced meal, or at least some food to eat, and umm, as long as she's sitting with us having the meals with us.

THERAPIST: Well, you know that's a good start. You also know that she needs to recover the weight as quickly as possible. Chronic malnutrition is extremely hard on the body, and it reinforces the whole process. So, I would encourage you to find an approach which would encourage her to gain the weight at a reasonable rate. Because of the things that can happen . . . you may have met some of these young women . . . they hover between really not getting admitted, and being a good weight. And that's not a good thing, the body is incredibly malnourished, and the eating disorder becomes more and more entrenched with the style of being in the world, and all the damage to the bones and the muscles, and the other psychological issues, the preoccupation with calories and lack of ability to focus on other things, become even more pronounced. It's not a good pattern, (to Rhonda) you really need to get over that hurdle and into healthy weights so that you can go on with your life.

The therapist now tries to focus the parents once more by emphasizing just what the consequences of chronic starvation for Rhonda may be. He does this to mobilize the parents into taking the steps it will require to restore Rhonda's weight to normal. The therapist prepares to become more directive in the session regarding refeeding, as ample time has now transpired and the parents are not taking direct action to confront the eating-disordered behaviors. The therapist also repeats and reinforces some of the dire consequences of eating disorders from a health perspective. Although this was discussed in Session 1, it is important to keep reemphasizing these problems, as they seem to easily slip out of view for the family, leaving them unprepared for the action that they need to take to preserve their child's health.

MOTHER: One of the things I'm concerned about is when Rhonda can start her period, but I think it's somewhere around 100 pounds or so. If she's not at 100 pounds, then she wouldn't be able to start her period.

THERAPIST: Probably not.

MOTHER: So, you have another 10 pounds to go before you can start your period.

FATHER: I don't understand how that works because how does the body know, for a female, that you have to be a certain weight.

THERAPIST: Because women need to be well nourished in order to have menses. The purpose behind having menses is that you're capable of having a child. So the idea here is that your body is strong and healthy enough to grow. To nurture an infant requires you have a certain amount of body weight. That's how your body knows, and what happens is that the whole cycle, the whole menstrual cycle, is based on a set of hormonal responses that tell your body you're strong and healthy. That's one of the reasons the bones are affected. Certain hormones are produced during the menstrual cycle which lead to the deposition of calcium in the bones. All of that fits together as a single piece in a woman's body. So basically in puberty, girls put on weight because they're fertile. Your body would be able to sustain itself with an infant or fetus in your body. And you need to have that, to have your whole body healthy. It's all one piece. You can't, for example, say, "I don't want a fetus so it doesn't matter." Because all the hormonal cycles which support the rest, the thyroid, the bone, fit together.

The therapist continues to educate the parents and Rhonda about the health consequences of the disorder and to do so clearly and with as little medical jargon as possible.

MOTHER: I was asking questions to our gynecologist, because I was saying on Friday that I was concerned about Rhonda not having a period so that's why we took her to the gynecologist. And sometimes they can give you a shot to induce menstrual cycles, that's when she suspected an eating disorder.

THERAPIST: That's artificial.

MOTHER: Yeah, but she said that in order to produce enough estrogen to start the cycle you need a certain amount of body fat. I was just flabbergasted in the hospital when the nutritionist told Rhonda that she had like only 9% body fat.

THERAPIST: What do you think it should be?

The therapist does not test the parents' knowledge but rather helps them along to learn more about the illness. But more important, he slowly demonstrates to the parents how starved their daughter is, in the hope that they become sufficiently alarmed to take action against the starvation.

MOTHER: About 20 to 25, I think.

FATHER: Oh, you're kidding. Oh, I didn't know that. 20 to 25!

THERAPIST: 18 to 25. That's how far down she was.

FATHER: So, she was exactly half of the minimum.

MOTHER: Or less.

FATHER: Okay, so what you're saying is that it should be done quickly.

THERAPIST: It should be at a safe rate, now that Rhonda is out of the hospital. When you're in the hospital, you know, she's on bed rest, so she needed to go very slow, because they don't want to overwhelm the heart with fluid suddenly. Now that she's out of the hospital, she can gain weight at a reasonable rate.

MOTHER: Well, Rhonda is really cognizant of eating good foods, a lot of carbohydrates, vegetables, fruits. She hasn't been eating much fruits lately.

THERAPIST: She's knowledgeable about food, I can tell.

FATHER: And what happens if she doesn't? We always get the same thing. "I'm not hungry, I'm full."

The therapist specifically addresses the parents now, and after convincing them of the seriousness of the illness for their daughter, he turns to them to address them directly about what needs to be eaten here and now. Also, the parents should explore here, with the therapist's support, ways to get Rhonda to eat as much as is reasonably required to gain weight.

THERAPIST: Do you think she should eat more now?

MOTHER: Definitely.

FATHER: Yes.

THERAPIST: Can you figure out a way to help her?

FATHER: Well, normally what we'll do at home is, we'll sit there with her and give her more time to eat it.

THERAPIST: (to Rhonda) Okay, well, you're here, does that work?

FATHER: Are you listening? C'mon, Rhonda.

RHONDA: I'm listening.

THERAPIST: She's definitely listening.
          (Laughter)

FATHER: I can't believe she drank this whole bottle.

THERAPIST: What is that?

FATHER: It's Select Clear, carbonated.

THERAPIST: I think the idea is that fills her up.

FATHER: You mean the liquid?

THERAPIST: Makes you full, right?

RHONDA: (nodding)

FATHER: Oh, so that's the trick, and there are no calories? Total fat zero.

THERAPIST: If that was a thing of cream, you know, a creamy milkshake . . . that would have been good, she would have gotten some calories. Those are sort of empty, empty filling-up fluids. Why did you buy the diet? I also noticed that you have Lay's potato chips, not diet. She has fat free potato chips.

RHONDA: I didn't ask for any particular one.

MOTHER: She didn't ask for this.

FATHER: Because she wouldn't have eaten it if I would have got her something else, and she didn't eat it that way anyway.

The parents are understandably reluctant to tackle the eating disorder, as is clear from this interaction—they would rather provide the patient with low-fat or fat-free food. The therapist's task is to get the parents to rely on foods that will help someone who is starved gain weight. If there have to be discussions about food with the patient, they should rather be about pasta with cream sauce as opposed to fat-free yogurt. The therapist also begins to be more instructive here, that is, to help the parents find ways to succeed in getting their daughter to eat as much as they think she ought to. Although the therapist confronts the parents on their decisions in the preceding exchanges, the tone is supportive, not accusatory. The therapist begins more active coaching in the exchanges that follow. This coaching begins with verbal suggestions, then proceeds to physical gestures, and finally to active coaching from behind the parents' chairs.

THERAPIST: Well, you know she needs the fat right?

MOTHER: Yeah, here (*handing her the regular bag of chips*).

FATHER: It's the same thing with yogurt that she gets at home, because she loves yogurt, it's the fat free.

THERAPIST: Maybe you could do more that just handing her the bag? Maybe you (*to the parents*) could think of something more to do?

RHONDA: I never, like, I've never been, I don't think, a real soda drinker.

FATHER: You could eat your sandwich. You ate the bigger half first, so that will be easier to get down.

MOTHER: Well, I told her, too, it should be a cinch out of the hospital. Because in the hospital she was given only a half hour to eat her meals except for dinner, which was 45 minutes. But she could take longer to eat.

THERAPIST: Well, let me also say that I think you should also think about that, too. You can't sit 3 hours at a dinner. That's another thing I'm going to ask you to take on. The goal is to eat a reasonable amount of calories in a reasonable amount of time. She's got to learn to manage that. She used to be able to do that, it's the illness that has kept her from being able to do that. She needs to be able to eat normally again. You taught her how to do that when she was little. You taught her how to do it. What has she learned? It sounds like many things you do as a family at dinner are really healthy, you sit and you enjoy it together and so forth. So now, she's gotten out of the loop, you got to get her back into the loop.

RHONDA: This morning, like, this morning, I had a muffin and stuff, but I went into the cupboards so I could pick at some cereal, because I had a Power Bar and I also had a muffin. And I went to pick at some cereal, I also had a Boost a little later on. But, I picked at it.

THERAPIST: (*encouraging the parents to be more active and pointing at the chips*) If you don't want to open them, there's some over there.

MOTHER: Is there any left in here?

FATHER: Not many. Take a couple.

THERAPIST: We're listening to you, but I want you to focus on getting her to eat.

RHONDA: I went back in the candy thing and I had a couple pieces of candy, because I hadn't had candy.

THERAPIST: So it wasn't a binge? You didn't feel it was a binge?

RHONDA: Well, I had like more than a couple pieces, but then I felt guilty after that.

THERAPIST: Did you purge after?

RHONDA: No. But I felt guilty. Because if you do it will show up on your vital signs.

THERAPIST: (*to Rhonda*) So, why are you eating that sandwich?

FATHER: I know why she is, so she wouldn't have to get into the potato chips.

MOTHER: But you love food, you enjoy food. You had a good time on Sunday. She had three big croissants, I mean they were delicious.

FATHER: And she didn't eat slow either. No, she ate like a normal person would eat, and she got up and she got another plate.

MOTHER: You know, potatoes, salad, and stuff.

FATHER: That's why it kind of surprised me.

THERAPIST: Why are you eating that sandwich?

RHONDA: Because I like it.

THERAPIST: Do you want to eat it?

RHONDA: Yeah.

THERAPIST: Do you, really?

RHONDA: Yeah.

The therapist tries to establish what motivated the patient to eat. Sometimes the patient may eat, not because of the parents' pressure but rather to thwart their attempt to feel empowered. The therapist wants to avoid this, if possible. To do so, he may encourage the patient at the onset of the meal (albeit paradoxically) to resist her parents' attempts at getting her to eat. The aim is to provide the parents with an opportunity to succeed in defeating the eating disorder.

THERAPIST: Okay, if you're choosing to eat, I want to know, because you're still eating it.

FATHER: And she told us the other night that she really loves food. And that's half the battle, I think.

THERAPIST: Rhonda, I have to just cut in here because I kind of heard you under your breath say, when your dad said, "I want you to eat that half sandwich," and you said "Not now."

FATHER: I heard it, too.
      (*Laughter*)

RHONDA: Well, if you gave me that choice, then, I mean. . . .

MOTHER: You give in easily.

RHONDA: It wouldn't be exactly. . . .

MOTHER: Would you eat it later when we go home?

Supporting the Daughter's Autonomy and Adolescent Development*

Because there are no siblings, the therapist must take a more active and supportive role in this particular family in relation to the daughter. This can be tricky for the therapist, as he must balance actively encouraging the parents to take on the illness while more directly supporting

*As there are no siblings in this family, this maneuver is adjusted to take this into account.

the resistance of the patient at times. To do this in this type of family requires a rather constant movement back and forth on the therapist's part between empowering the parents and supporting the adolescent. In a family with siblings present, the therapist would encourage the siblings to form an alliance that supports the patient rather than having to take this on himself.

THERAPIST: Here's my point: I want you to eat it because it's good for you nutritionally, and I know there's a part of you that wants not to eat it, and I don't want that part of you just to pretend. Okay? It doesn't help us to do this work if you're going to pretend to go along with it. And some of what you did before, you described it very eloquently today, you said "I would eat with my parents, and then I would go upstairs and purge." That was a way of kind of pretending to go along with it. And that's because you love your parents, and you don't want to make them angry. But you've got to get in there with this, you've got to, you can't pretend. Otherwise, you and they won't be able to work it out, they've got to know what they're up against, and they've still got to fight it. Does this make sense to you?

RHONDA: Yeah, but it's still, it's not easy to, because if they tell me to go eat something, it's not easy to just go in there and eat it and not still have the thought "I don't want to eat this."

THERAPIST: You can still have that thought.

RHONDA: I mean I always have that thought, "I don't want to eat this," but I'm eating it, because if I don't it will obviously, obviously show up somewhere, you know, vital signs.

THERAPIST: I want that part of you that's a fighter, and creative. You know, you showed some real ingenuity here, fooled your parents who know you very well, on a few occasions. I want that applied to other areas of your life. I don't want that squashed, I want to be clear about that. I don't want that independence, that creativity, that part of you that is your own person squashed, I don't want that. So that's not the part to struggle against, I just want you to apply it in a healthier way. But, right now, I want to know if you want to eat that sandwich because your parents want you to or not.

As pointed out earlier, the therapist wants to prevent the patient from "going along" and thereby denying the parents the opportunity to learn how to struggle effectively with the eating disorder.

RHONDA: If they want me to, I'll eat it.

FATHER: We'd love you to eat that sandwich.

RHONDA: If you want me to.

FATHER: We wish you would.

THERAPIST: Now, I want you to eat it only if you really want to.

RHONDA: I really don't want to eat it.

MOTHER: You really don't want to eat it?

RHONDA: Because of what I ate this morning.

THERAPIST: A muffin?

RHONDA: The muffin, Boost, candy, and a Power Bar.

FATHER: Total, if you add up all those calories, that's not enough.

RHONDA: It's about 1,500.

FATHER: What you ate?

RHONDA: Yeah.

FATHER: Without the sandwich?

RHONDA: It was about 1,500 or more.

MOTHER: Including right here?

FATHER: No, she's saying without the sandwich.

RHONDA: I'm saying without the sandwich.

MOTHER: So, 1,500 until dinner time, right?

RHONDA: 1,500 or 1,600.

FATHER: With a Power Bar and a muffin, and a Boost.

RHONDA: Because those little muffins are like 300 or 400 calories, because from the ones we had in the hospital, they were high.

FATHER: They were like 240 or 260.

RHONDA: 370.

FATHER: Were they that size?

RHONDA: Smaller.

MOTHER: So let's say the muffin could be 300. So with 300, and the Boost 240, and the Power Bar 230, right?

RHONDA: Yeah.

MOTHER: That's not even 1,000.

RHONDA: What do you mean, it's not even 1,000? I had all that candy.

MOTHER: Oh, the candy, oh, the little pieces of candy.

FATHER: So, we really shouldn't be buying anything that's fat free. I know we shouldn't be.

THERAPIST: No.

The therapist tries to prevent the parents from entering a debate about the caloric value of foods with their daughter. It may be all right to discuss that between themselves, but they should avoid getting stuck with their daughter in this way. Decisions about food should be in the parental domain.

MOTHER: Maybe for me it's okay.

FATHER: Would anybody like this half? I didn't touch it.

THERAPIST: Thank you. No, I really don't want to eat, this is your, your meal. But, maybe Rhonda will eat it tomorrow.

MOTHER: For lunch.

THERAPIST: So, I want to make clear what happened here. We're almost out of time. Did you follow what happened, you ate a little bit and you fought a little bit, right, more than you wanted? You ate a little more than you wanted. And you helped her do it. You can do it, you can help her.

RHONDA: But I also ate that because you were here.

THERAPIST: You mean I need to be at your house? For all the meals? (*Laughter*)

MOTHER: Maybe in spirit.

THERAPIST: Well, if that's what you need to imagine, I'm there, every single meal. And I'm certainly behind helping you, because I want you to get well.

RHONDA: Because what I do, I figure in advance what I'm going to eat that day. What I think I'm going to eat, and then I add in some calories in case I eat something unexpectedly. Like today, I figured it was like 1,500 or 1,600, and so I went with 1,600, plus I figured like 300 for the half a sandwich, so about 1,900.

MOTHER: The other one, with the blue cap, is sodium free, caffeine free, but it does have calories. So you can get the one with calories.

RHONDA: No, it's not sodium free, because that's where the calories come from, it's because it has sugar in it, that's why.

Again, the therapist encourages the parents to make food decisions and to remove debate about fat-free foods from their discussions. The therapist ends the session by congratulating the parents on their efforts in order to bolster their confidence in their ability to address the eating disorder effectively.

THERAPIST: Remember, Rhonda knows a lot about food.

MOTHER: She's going to manipulate our minds, our psyches.

Closing the Session

THERAPIST: No, she just knows, she's learned it. You just need to know that you know something about it, too, and you know what it's going to take. You knew that wasn't the one with calories. You knew what she was going to eat and what she wasn't. But you did as a family eat today and began working on the problems that anorexia has brought to the family. It seems to me that you have a lot of good skills going into this struggle and are learning a lot about how anorexia makes Rhonda behave. Those will all be helpful as you move ahead in making sure that Rhonda eats better.

So we will meet next Friday?

8

The Remainder of Phase I
(Sessions 3–10)

Most of the remainder of this phase is characterized by the therapist's attempts to bring the patient's food intake under parental control by expanding, reinforcing, and repeating some of the tasks initiated at the beginning of therapy. What the therapist has to achieve here, in addition to continuing the work begun in Sessions 1 and 2 is to review with the parents, on a regular basis, their attempts at refeeding the patient and to systematically advise the parents how to proceed in curtailing the influence of the eating disorder. Sessions are characterized by a considerable degree of repetition, as the therapist may go over the same steps week after week to get the parents to become consistent in their management of the patient's eating behavior and the eating disorder's attempt to defeat these efforts.

Unlike the more structured nature of the first two meetings, the following sessions may seem less systematically organized and may not follow a prespecified order. However, a combination of the following three goals will apply to almost every session until the conclusion of Phase I of treatment.

There are three goals for these treatment sessions:

- To keep the family focused on the eating disorder.
- To help the parents take charge of their daughter's eating.
- To mobilize siblings to support the patient.

In order to accomplish these goals, the following interventions will be appropriate to consider during the remainder of treatment for Phase I:

1. Weighing the patient at the beginning of each session.
2. Directing, redirecting, and focusing the therapeutic discussion on food and eating behaviors and their management until food, eating, and weight behaviors and concerns are relieved.
3. Discussing, supporting, and helping the parental dyad's efforts at refeeding.
4. Discussing, supporting, and helping the family to evaluate efforts of siblings to help their affected sister.
5. Continuing to modify parental and sibling criticisms.
6. Continuing to distinguish the adolescent patient and her interests from those of AN.
7. Closing all sessions with a recounting of progress.

These goals will be applied in Sessions 3 through 10 in any order, with their momentary applicability or appropriateness determined by the family's response to the initial interventions (Sessions 1 and 2). For the purpose of clarification, however, we will outline a description of each goal separately, even though in practice they may overlap to a considerable degree. Patients may require a range of sessions for completion of Phase I, sometimes as few as two to three additional sessions to as many as 10 or more.

Weighing the Patient at the Beginning of Each Session

Why

As in the first two sessions, weighing the patient is an important opportunity to assess the patient and her progress. It is also an opportunity to continue to build some rapport with her. Because the parents are being encouraged by the therapist to actively refeed her, often against her wishes, it may be that the remainder of Phase I is a trial of the relationship between the therapist and the patient. It is helpful to be as sympathetic and open to the patient as possible during these brief weighing periods. At these weighing periods, it is also sometimes useful to ask the adolescent specifically whether there may be certain issues she would like the therapist to put forward in the session.

The pattern of weight gain can be quite variable. In one family, who readily take up the task of refeeding and who figure out quickly how to accomplish this, weight gain may occur swiftly. On the other hand, many families struggle with a variety of issues that prevent them from achieving the refeeding of their starving daughter or son. For example, parents may have trouble working together. They may disagree on the strategy to employ. One of them may not make it a priority to assist with refeeding. Parents may try to avoid taking their daughter out of school, even though she is not eating, because they so value her accomplishments there. Siblings may undermine their ill brother or sister by becoming unruly in some manner themselves. Most often, the parents are extremely reluctant to take on the strong will of the child with AN because they know what they are up against and do not want to face this challenge. In some cases, one parent may be overinvolved with the accomplishments of their affected son or daughter and be unwilling to challenge their behaviors. For example, one mother so wanted her daughter to dance in a particular ballet that she continued to take her to class even after it was evident that her daughter was continuing to become dangerously malnourished. For all of these reasons and many more like them, the weight-gain course may be quite variable. In general, however, by Sessions 5 and 6 a pattern that suggests that the parents are beginning to be successful should be evident. If it is not, the therapist should be concerned that some aspect of the interventions are not being used by the family or that one of the types of problems discussed previously is preventing progress.

How

The therapist's own resilience in staying with the eating-disorder symptoms will send a powerful message to the parents that, for now, this is the focus of treatment. The therapist starts every session by first recording the patient's weight and carefully plotting it on a weight chart. Weight progress, or lack thereof, is shared with the entire family. Some time should be spent explaining to the parents how the patient's weight compares with those of her peers, and the therapist should either congratulate them when progress has been made or sympathize when there has been no progress. At this early stage of treatment, the therapist should continue to point out just how dangerously underweight the patient is (regardless of initial weight gain) so as to keep the parents focused on the task at hand. It may be helpful to ask the parents to bring in family photographs to get a view of the patient's normal body shape. This helps the parents to visualize a healthy picture of their daughter and to prevent them from accepting the status quo. Parents often take premature comfort from initial weight gain and begin to relax their vigilance. The therapist should be alert to this probability and continue to model his or her concern for the patient's physical and mental state and to emphasize the urgency of continuing weight gain.

Directing, Redirecting, and Focusing the Therapeutic Discussion on Food and Eating Behaviors and Their Management until Food, Eating, and Weight Behaviors and Concerns Are Relieved

Why

As stated before, the primary challenge for the parents during Phase I of treatment is to engage successfully in the task of refeeding their anorexic daughter. Whereas initially the therapist may have to work hard to convince the parents that drastic action is required, for the remainder of Phase 1, in most instances, the therapist has to keep the family focused on the eating disorder. Parents may become fatigued or the patient may gain weight initially, creating the illusion that the immediate crisis has been removed. Because AN can become intractable and because it can be wearing to continue to confront, therapists and families alike may be tempted to relax their efforts too soon. However, this would be an error, as a mind that is preoccupied with AN thoughts usually takes every opportunity to reassert itself.

How

The usual result of Session 3 is the gain of more control by the parents, although weight gain may not yet be evident. Dehydrated patients may be one exception, as they may quickly gain several pounds after the first visit. Regardless of weight gain, the therapist may provide basic dietary instructions and coach the parents in terms of their refeeding skills from Session 3 onward. This is done by eliciting from the family their large, but often unused, store of knowledge about what constitutes healthy eating and sufficient amounts of high-caloric foods suitable for a starving person, as well as their particular understanding of their child. Parents soon become inventive and begin to create high-density meals. Although discussions about diet should be discouraged, when they do occur, the aim is to encourage the parents to debate the value of a meal of 1,000 calories or more instead of getting locked into unproductive and futile arguments with their daughter about the negligible caloric content of a salad of lettuce leaves or a fat-free yogurt. The emphasis on gaining weight should be placed in the overall context of achieving a weight that the patient's healthy body "knows is right," that is, through a return of healthy skin and hair, return of menses, and an increase in bone density. In other words, the therapist should see weight gain less in term of "norms" or numbers on a scale and more in terms of a particular patient's health. The therapist should refrain from setting a specific target weight. Instead, the goal of a healthy body should be used to guide the patient toward a healthy weight. This weight is essentially a range that the patient can sustain without undue dieting and, if female, one at which menses is comfortably maintained.

After the family meal, feeding will remain a preoccupation for the next several sessions, even when the patient is gaining weight under the new regimen. The therapist has to insist that the parents remain relentless until they are convinced that the patient clearly understands that she will not be able to return to anorexic behavior while a part of the parents' household. Consequently, the therapist will stress the need for regular, dietetically balanced food intake, while vegetarianism may be temporarily suspended. Other symptoms (such as binge eating and purging) should also be subject to strict parental control. As is the case with dietary control, this control should be emphasized as a temporary measure. The intention is for the parents to demonstrate that they can achieve control and, if necessary, remove the possibility of their daughter being able to make herself sick again. This may include keeping their daughter occupied after a meal (e.g., watching a favorite movie on television), supervised bathroom visits, locking the kitchen if possible, and so forth. It may also include visiting local pharmacies to inform them of the possibility that their daughter is abusing laxatives and to ask that they be contacted if she attempts to purchase them.

Once the weight chart has been explained and discussed, the therapist should carefully review events surrounding eating during the past week. The family's strategies for bringing about weight gain should dominate discussions, especially in the absence of significant symptomatic improvements. The therapist will ask each parent, the patient, and her siblings to tell him or her how the past week has been and how they have gone about the task of refeeding. The therapist should discourage broad statements such as, "it's been an okay week," or "it was difficult." Instead, he or she will turn to each parent separately and ask them to relay in great detail what happened at mealtimes and, in the same style of circular questioning outlined before, check with every family member in turn whether that is also the way they would describe events. Discrepancies should be lingered over, and the therapist should search for clarification. The therapist should be able to construct a clear picture of what happens at mealtimes, as well as between mealtimes, so that he or she can carefully select those steps parents have taken that should be reinforced and those that should be discouraged. For example, one family was worried because their daughter consumed most of her food in the evening. The daughter explained that she felt uncomfortable eating in front of her friends. As this patient was eating well and gaining weight, the family was encouraged to delay this struggle until their daughter was more recovered. Although the therapist no longer has the therapeutic advantage of having the family eat a picnic lunch in his or her office, which enabled him or her to intervene directly to reinforce or correct certain behaviors, he or she should use these initial sessions that follow the family meal to carefully bolster the parents in their knowledge of high-density meals, to bring about healthy eating, and to discourage any behaviors that may impede this process.

Discussing, Supporting, and Helping the Parental Dyad's Efforts at Refeeding

Why

One of the most important aspects of this treatment at this particular juncture is the therapist ensuring that the parents are working together as a team. The parents' success in refeeding their daughter can often directly be attributed to their ability to work as a team in this process. Because the aim of the therapy is develop, enrich, and support the parents in their efforts to care for their ill adolescent, the ability of the therapist to provide assistance in this is crucial. At the same time, the therapist may be tempted to "take over" the parental role by directing or overcontrolling the refeeding process. This hazard should be avoided, because the ultimate message of the therapy is that the family, not the therapist, is the major resource for recovery.

How

The therapist might have to emphasize to the parents that although he or she understands and respects that they (the parents) may have differences of opinion, as many couples may have, parents cannot afford to differ at all in how they should refeed their daughter. The therapist should exercise extreme vigilance in checking with the parents on a weekly basis as to how they are doing in this regard. In carefully reviewing their attempts at refeeding as described previously, the therapist also checks with everyone on how the parents are doing as a team. The therapist makes it a point to address the parents as "the authoritative team" to reinforce for them that they are indeed in charge. Consistently addressing the parents as the key decision makers in relation to their daughter's health matters also reinforces for their daughter and her siblings that the parents are in charge in this arena. Making decisions jointly as a couple may in fact be uncharted territory for some parents. Reminding the parents that they should work together and that they should be "on the same page, on the same line, and on the same word, at all times when it comes to their daughter's eating" should be done at several time points in this early part of treatment.

Discussing, Supporting, and Helping the Family to Evaluate Efforts of Siblings to Help Their Affected Sister

Why

To reinforce healthy cross-generational boundaries and to prevent the siblings from interfering with the parents' task of refeeding, consistent support of the patient by her siblings should be encouraged. Healthy boundaries between the siblings and their parents make the parents' immediate task less difficult, while also preparing the groundwork for successful resolution of the eating disorder and the launching of a healthy adolescent into young adulthood.

How

Similar to the stated aim for this part of Phase I, the therapist should be consistent in his or her encouragement of the siblings not to interfere with their parents' task but rather to support their sister through this ordeal. The therapist will say to the siblings, "While your parents make every effort to fight your sister's illness and nourish her back to health, she will think that they are being awful to her and she will need to be able to tell someone just how bad things are for her; that is, she will need someone like yourselves who could listen to her complaints. She will also need you to comfort her when she feels that things are too rough for her and she gets too scared about eating and weight gain."

Realigning the patient with her siblings may be an arduous process, as the eating disorder may have caused the patient to isolate herself from her siblings or peers over a protracted period of time. Also, extricating the adolescent from an overinvolved relationship with one or both parents may prove to be equally difficult. However, the therapist should be consistent in his or her monitoring of the siblings' efforts to involve their sister in their activities and of the ways they have found to be supportive of her during this process of refeeding. This support will obviously vary depending on the relationship that existed between the siblings prior to the onset of the illness. Verbal support of the patient should be encouraged, as well as providing the adolescent the opportunity to express her sadness, frustration, or anger. It is important for the adolescent to feel that she has an ally during this process of refeeding. In some cases, the adolescent may have only one sibling who is much younger than she is, or she may in fact be an only child. A younger brother or sister may not be capable of providing verbal comfort to the adolescent. However, the therapist could suggest that the younger sibling give his or her sister a couple of hugs every day in order to reassure her that he or she is trying to be comforting or to be supportive. This process is, of course, more complicated when the adolescent does not have any siblings. The therapist should then take careful note of the relationship the patient has with her peers or that she may have had prior to the onset of the illness. This is done so that the therapist may help the parents to identify suitable social activities outside the family home through which the adolescent can meet and spend time with her peers. The aim here is the same as with siblings, that is, an opportunity for the adolescent to become more aligned with her age group and to feel supported through this period of time.

The therapist will want to discourage siblings from rushing to their parents' aid in feeding the patient or attempting to deter them from pursuing their task of refeeding the patient. In addition to explaining to the family that the job of refeeding belongs to the parents and that supporting and comforting the patient during this time are the tasks of the brothers and sisters, the therapist should reinforce the siblings in this role throughout treatment. For instance, efforts by siblings to jump to the parents' rescue while they (the parents) try to get the patient to eat more or to discourage parents from pushing too hard, should be prevented. The therapist should ensure that the siblings are relegated to the status of observers in this process. Groundwork for this maneuver is prepared during Sessions 1 and 2. For instance, during the family meal the therapist might have had a firsthand opportunity to observe whether siblings are inclined to interfere with the parents' refeeding attempts. At that time also the therapist may have had the first opportunity to intervene directly, by instructing a sibling *not* to try to help the parents or *not* to try to discourage the parents in their efforts. For the remainder of this phase of treatment, the therapist should take a detailed account of how the family, and the siblings in particular, went about their efforts during the past week to make sure that the patient ate (the parents' task) and that she could turn to her siblings for support.

Continuing to Modify Parental and Sibling Criticisms

Why

It has been shown that parental criticism of the anorexic offspring can have a negative impact on the family's ability to remain in treatment, as well as on the eventual outcome in treatment. Consequently, it is of great importance to address parental criticism. We believe these criticisms are due to parental guilt about the eating disorder or to a reaction to the eating disorder symptoms per se, or may be indications of a poor premorbid relationship between the adolescent and her parents. Sessions in this part of treatment are therefore characterized by attempting to absolve the parents from the responsibility of causing the illness and by complimenting them as much as possible on the positive aspects of their parenting of their children.

How

We have already made mention of the fact that modeling by the therapist of an uncritical acceptance of the patient is an essential therapeutic task. This is achieved in part by externalizing the illness; that is, the therapist must convince the parents that most of the patient's behaviors in regard to eating are in fact outside of her control and that it is the illness that has overtaken her behavior in this respect. In other words, the therapist must consistently point to the fact that the patient cannot be identified with the illness. Doing this helps to foster an understanding of the patient's behavior and to reduce any parental criticism of the patient. Changing parents' behavior in this regard can be difficult, but persistence on the therapist's behalf may pay dividends in the end. For instance, some parents may say, in response to anorexic behaviors from their daughter, "She is making it so difficult for us, we make an effort to get the foods she likes, and then we catch her trying to throw it in the trash." Or, "We are desperate now, because if we just turn our backs for a second, she'll give her food to the dog, or stick it in her pockets." Or, "I've had it with X, I have to be with her 24 hours a day, because if I dare let her out of my sight, she's up and down the stairs exercising." These examples demonstrate that in all three cases the anorexic behaviors have been identified with the patient. Another way of reading or understanding these passages is to hear the parent's unspoken words: "I am trying my best, and just look how deceitful or ungrateful our daughter is." As pointed out before, parental anger, frustration, or criticism can have deleterious consequences for the successful resolution of the eating disorder.

The therapist can help counteract the impact of comments such as these in several ways. First, he or she has made an effort in the first couple of sessions to separate the illness from the adolescent, thereby demonstrating to the parents the perception that this disorder "has come into your daughter's life and has overtaken her feelings, thoughts, and behaviors as far as food, eating, and body weight are concerned. It is the eating disorder that is making your daughter behave in ways that you have not associated with X. I am sure X has been a good child and wouldn't necessarily lie to you or act in other deceptive ways, such as hiding food. However, this illness is extremely powerful, and because it has overtaken X's behaviors in so many ways, it is the eating disorder we observe when food is hidden, or when X puts up a fight to resist your efforts at refeeding." Second, the therapist should be consistent in her or his efforts during ensuing sessions to refer to symptomatic behaviors as "that's the illness," or "it's the anorexia talking," and to say such things as, "I wonder what the healthy X may be thinking about," or "I am sure if the healthy X was in charge, then . . . ," when he or she wants to draw a clear distinction between these two parts of the struggling adolescent. Third, the therapist should make every effort to correct the parents throughout this part of treatment at every juncture when a family member says something that identifies the illness with the patient; for example, "I know you are very concerned about your daughter/sister, especially when you see her behave in ways you are shocked by, or disapprove of. However, it is important that we remember that it is the anorexia that is in charge and that is influencing X to behave in this way. Therefore, we all have to work very hard so that we can help diminish the power of this illness so that X's healthy part can flourish again." In guiding the parents through this difficult period, the therapist should remember that families have very different ways of parenting and different circumstances that will influence how this process is worked through. It is important to remember that each family should be encouraged to work out for themselves how best to refeed their anorexic child.

Continuing to Distinguish the Adolescent Patient and Her Interests from Those of Anorexia Nervosa

Why

As discussed in the description of the Session 1 intervention, it is important that the therapist and the family keep in mind that they are struggling to combat the effects of AN and not the independent thinking and will of a developing adolescent person. If the therapist fails to keep this idea a focused aspect of the treatment during this phase, the hope for developing an alliance with the patient is greatly diminished and her resistance to the treatment enhanced.

How

Again, this intervention is discussed in the Session 1 description. However, as Phase I continues, the therapist may stress the need to recognize that more of the effort of eating is safely being taken up by the healthy part of the patient. This can be done by saying things such as, "It seems to me that your parents reported that they needed to encourage you less to eat and that you are more interested in fighting back AN yourself," or, alternatively, asking something like, "As you have been progressing you are taking more of your life back. Have you noticed that your thoughts are less preoccupied by food and weight?" The therapist may ask the patient to gauge her progress figuratively; for example, by drawing a Venn diagram that shows how much of herself remains preoccupied by AN (see Figure 8.1). At least part of every session should be devoted to these times of observations, questions, and assessments.

Review Progress with Treatment Team

As was the case for Sessions 1 and 2, the lead therapist should continue to review each treatment session with the rest of the team for the remainder of Phase I. At the end of each session, the following information should be conveyed to the treatment and consultation team: the patient's weight progress, development of any new symptoms (e.g., purging, overexercise, etc.), new diagnostic concerns (e.g., anxiety disorder, depression, suicidality, etc.), and on overall sense of the family's progress with the illness. Any problems between team members (i.e., medical team not informing parents of progress or concerns) should be discussed.

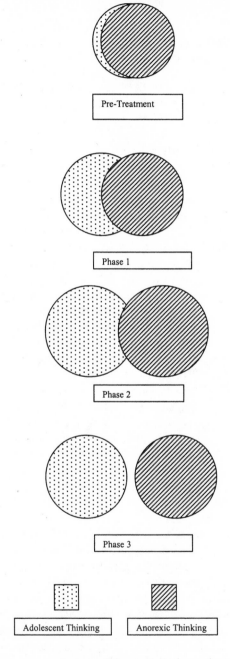

FIGURE 8.1. Diagram comparing adolescent's independent thinking to thoughts and behaviors that result from AN.

Common Questions for Sessions 3–10

What kind of detail about how the week progressed should be solicited from the parents?

In the early part of Phase I of treatment, after the therapist has opened the session with a review of the patient's weight, he or she should always review with the family in considerable detail how the past week has been. For instance, "Could you tell me exactly how things went for you this week in your attempts to restore X's weight? In so doing, I want you to tell me very specifically how a difficult meal went, how you decided on the amount of food you gave X, exactly how much and what kinds of food you presented to her, and how you tried to get her to eat this meal." In so doing, the therapist may interrupt the parents frequently in attempt to gain an exact picture of this process. A parent may say, "We gave her some pasta and a salad, and . . . ," and the therapist may say, "How did you decide on pasta, and exactly how much did you think would help her gain the weight she needs to put on, and . . . ?" In other words, as the parents give their account of events, the therapist wants to get a complete picture, linger over inconsistencies, and engage the parents to try and clarify their differences in accounting the events of the past week. The therapist takes very careful note of the steps the parents may have taken that might not have helped X to progress. For instance, one parent may say that he or she put a plate of pasta in front of X, whereas the other parent notes that the portion size was not sufficient or perhaps too much. At such a point the therapist ought to explore with the parents how they decided on the portion size. If the decision was not made as a team, the therapist should encourage them to approach similar events in the week to come differently. By the time the adolescent is presented with a plate of food, both parents should have agreed beforehand on the amount of food and on how they will "stick it out" in their attempts to get X to eat her meal. Likewise, the therapist should also take note of the steps the parents have taken that do seem to have paid off and to make sure to praise them and reinforce their efforts. Throughout this process, the therapist reinforces the parents' own strengths and parenting skills and encourages them to delve into their own reservoirs of knowledge about how to raise their children in general and how to feed someone in their family who is starving. As mentioned earlier, each family has to work out the way to refeed their daughter that works best for them. That should not discourage the therapist from suggesting to the parents that they should not promote behaviors such as calorie counting or get bogged down in "anorexic debate," that is, arguing with their adolescent daughter at length about the relative merits of a salad as opposed to a pasta with a cream sauce. The parents sometimes need to hear repeatedly that buying food, preparing food, and deciding what and how much food their daughter should eat should be their decision only. While parents are wrestling with issues such as whether they should have X attend school for now or not or how to deal with temper tantrums or competition between the patient and siblings, the therapist should allow them to work out how to cope with these dilemmas. Reminding them of their responsibility as a team, however, remains crucial.

How can the adolescent be aligned with peers when there are no siblings?

It is not uncommon for an adolescent to be an only child or perhaps the youngest child whose siblings have already moved out of the parental home. In both instances, the therapist works only with the parents and their anorexic offspring. We emphasized the process of aligning the adolescent with her peers earlier in this chapter. The therapist faces a challenge here in that, although it would be helpful to mobilize siblings to provide the patient with comfort and reintegration into appropriate adolescent life, this may not be possible. The only alternative the parents have is to encourage the patient to spend time with her peers at the opportune moments. For instance, while the parents are still struggling with getting the adolescent to eat sufficient amounts to reverse the self-starvation, it may not be advisable to encourage them to let X spend considerable amounts of time outside their supervision, especially during mealtimes. The parents should be encouraged though, to work out a way for their daughter to become more integrated with her peers, albeit gradually, especially once she returns to school. This can be done by having friends come over to the patient's house or by the patient's participation in some activities that take place outside of mealtimes and are time limited, for example, going to the movies with a school friend.

What if weight gain progresses well up to a certain point but then starts to plateau?

Some patients respond well initially and gain weight steadily to reach exercise weight. However, at a certain point—either when parents begin to drop their vigilance as they sense the crisis abating or at some arbitrary limit imposed by the patient, often before menstruation resumes—weight gain is halted. The therapist should use this opportunity to instill a "second crisis" in order to mobilize the parents once more to step up their efforts to refeed their daughter. It is often helpful to say something like, "Although it seems as if your daughter might be out of danger, this is not so. If she fails to continue the process of weight restoration, her malnutrition may become chronic, and this may lead to stunted growth, permanent infertility, osteoporosis, vertebral compression fractures, and so forth." From the patient's point of view, as she has gained some weight, she may experience a sense of loss, uncertainty, and a nostalgia for AN. This may be an important focus in Phase II of treatment.

What if the patient becomes more deceitful?

It is usually very difficult for parents to conceive of their daughter engaging in any deceitful behaviors, such as hiding weights on her body so as to record a higher weight at the hospital, or to discover, for instance, concealed laxatives or diuretics in the adolescent's room for the first time. Earlier in this chapter we discussed in detail the importance of the therapist in helping to separate the illness from the adolescent. When anorexic behaviors are reported in a session or when the family discovers such behaviors for the first time in a session, the therapist is afforded an ideal opportunity to model a noncritical way to explore these behaviors. For instance, when a therapist discovers that his or her patient has been hiding weights on her body at the time of weighing, he or she can calmly commiserate with the patient at the weighing, saying, "You must be so afraid of the consequences of gaining weight that your illness gets you to resort to such drastic efforts to convince us to back off. What a terrible struggle this must be for you." When the therapist convenes the meeting with the rest of the family, she or he, in a grave tone, should share the news about the hidden weights with the family in a way that clearly demonstrates to the patient that the therapist really understands her terrible anxiety and predicament. It should also show the parents that an angry response is *not* called for but rather one that commiserates with their daughter over the fear the illness creates that leads her to do such things. For instance, the therapist can say to the family, while facing the patient, "I have discovered with X today that the anorexia is so determined to fool us as far as X's weight is concerned that it got her to strap weights to her body so we can think she has gained weight." Turning to the parents, the therapist should add, "X is clearly in a predicament here, not having much control over these kinds of behaviors, and you will have to work out a way to help her out here so that we can diminish the power of this terrible illness." This discourse clearly illustrates how the therapist shows sympathy and understanding toward the patient while helping the parents to channel their frustrations toward the illness, not toward their daughter, and at the same time insisting that the parents take over the refeeding process.

How should the grandparents be involved?

Some families may live in close proximity to maternal and/or paternal grandparents. It is also often the case that the adolescent may spend significant time with her grandparents, for example, staying with grandparents after school until parents return home from work. The obvious question is whether and how these adults should be engaged in the adolescent's refeeding. The therapist should first learn from the family how involved the grandparents are in terms of their daughter's day-to-day care. If it appears as though considerable time is spent in the company of grandparents, then the therapist may want the grandparents to join the family for a session or two. This is especially important when the parents are not able to take any more time out of the office, when X's refeeding is still precarious, and when it is essential to have other responsible adults assist the parents in this potentially exhausting process. Once the therapist has an opportunity to meet with the grandparents, he or she may learn that the grandparents have an excellent understanding of the illness and of what is required to reverse the process of starvation. On the other hand, he or she may also learn that the adolescent's contact with her grandparents should be curtailed as long as she remains underweight, especially when it comes to mealtimes. This would be the case if the therapist comes to understand that the grandparents do not appreciate the seriousness of their granddaughter's condition and that the illness gets an opportunity to escape proper supervision, that is, that starvation is not curtailed in the presence of grandparents. It is therefore clear that the therapist should make a careful evaluation of (1) the time the adolescent normally spends with grandparents, (2) their understanding of the eating disorder and their ability to be as successful as the parents in preventing self-starvation, and (3) the level of exhaustion the parents may be experiencing and their need to have someone else rescue them from time to time.

How can a meddling team member be managed?

As we stated earlier, it is very important to assemble a multidisciplinary team for management of the eating disorder. It is also important that the team is "on the same line and on the same page" regarding the adolescent's treatment in the same way that the parents must be. It may sometimes happen that one team member tends to act on his or her own without regard for the overall plan that the primary therapist has put forward. This is especially the case among colleagues who do not have much experience operating as team members or who have not worked together with one another on prior occasions. It is therefore important, as indicated previously, for the lead therapist to remind other team members on a regular basis of the overall treatment goals and philosophy and of how the family has progressed in treatment. For instance, we believe it may be counterproductive to set forth a specific weight as a target to be reached in a certain amount of time. We choose instead to refer to a weight range or perhaps to think in terms of a menstruation weight. The therapist could use the fact that the patient is still not menstruating despite some significant weight gain as a way of reinvigorating the parents' efforts to return the patient's weight to a healthy menstruation weight. However, this tactic is obviously counterproductive if the adolescent's pediatrician believes that "menstruation is not that crucial at this time; many 15-year-olds don't menstruate." Proper communication between team members is therefore as important as the therapist's efforts to get the parents to work together.

How does parental psychopathology interfere with this therapy?

It is clear from our presentation so far that a great deal of commitment and stamina is required from parents in order to be successful in this treatment. It is inevitable that some parents may arrive at treatment with their own difficulties, such as an anxiety or mood disorder, which may potentially incapacitate them in their efforts to sustain focus and energy on the refeeding process. One way in which the therapist can buffer the impact of such circumstances is to refer that particular parent for individual support. For instance, when a parent arrives at treatment with a history of depression, it could be helpful to make sure that he or she has been evaluated by another professional with a view toward medication and psychotherapy support. Another way is to acknowledge that such events can potentially hamper parental efforts at refeeding and to have the parents work out a way between themselves to support one another. Although this book stresses at several junctures how important it is for parents to work as a team and to be in agreement about their way of refeeding their offspring, this does not necessarily imply that both parents should always be present at all refeeding episodes. We also stress that parents should work out for themselves how best to prevent their daughter from starving herself. Therefore, it is quite feasible that the healthier parent can relieve the distressed parent from time to time in the refeeding process, as long as they are always in agreement about how this process should be managed between them. Finally, we mentioned the role of grandparents and that in some instances they could be most helpful. If grandparents are available and the therapist and parents feel that they may be a good substitute for an unwell or exhausted parent from time to time, then arrangements ought to be made to have the grandparents help out with the refeeding process.

How does one manage highly critical or hostile families?

Studies by Eisler, Dare, Hodes, Russell, Dodge, and Le Grange (in press), and Le Grange, Eisler, Dare, and Russell (1992) suggest that children with AN who come from highly critical families may have a poorer prognosis than other families. As suggested previously, it is possible that such families may require a different form of family therapy—separated family therapy.

On the other hand, there is reason to explore ways of managing highly critical families in the whole-family therapy technique described in this manual. We believe that it is possible to approach highly critical families constructively. Our clinical experience has shown that modeling noncritical acceptance of the patient and her symptoms from the outset is the most helpful way to deal therapeutically with parental criticism toward the anorexic adolescent.

In addition to modeling noncritical behavior, the therapist can also notice critical comments made toward the patient or to the therapist about the patient, although more subtle rebukes of the patient or her symptoms may go astray. The therapist should not ignore these comments but must take note of them and help the parents to understand that it is the illness that makes their daughter resist their efforts, hide food, exercise excessively, and so forth. In other words, similar to the earlier strategy of externalizing the illness, the therapist should attempt to help the parents to understand that most of the patient's behaviors are outside her control. This effort may require considerable composure on the therapist's part. Support from the treatment team or the cotherapist can be helpful.

What may also be helpful at the outset of the treatment is for the therapist to work hard at absolving the parents from any blame for the eating disorder. In our experience, we have come to learn that parents burdened with guilt tend to be less successful in their efforts to help their daughter, and failure at this task may in fact exacerbate critical remarks toward the patient and her symptoms. Early and persistent education about the illness and its effects on the patient's thoughts and behaviors, even after significant weight restoration, can stave off criticism when parents see that their efforts do not swiftly bring on the desired effect of weight restoration and when psychopathology becomes evident in their offspring.

Once the patient and family have experienced some success, it is important that the therapist identify the impact of criticism on the progress or lack of progress that the patient is making. This requires that the therapist identify the issue of criticism and hostility without being critical or hostile him- or herself. Often these families are exquisitely sensitive to such criticism. The therapist can identify a problem without judgment and ask the family to explore it. The therapist guides the family through the problem to the core issue of the critical and hostile undercurrent that is impeding further progress.

It is helpful if the circumstance being examined for critical comment is both concrete and circumscribed. For example, the adolescent says she refused to eat for an entire day after a fight with her mother. This specific instance can serve as an example of the impact of the quality of interaction (critical) with the mother. At the same time, the therapist keeps the focus on this instance and does not actively interpret the hostility or criticism as the reason for not eating but encourages the family to see the impact of the interaction on the eating behavior.

Next, it is important that the therapist ask the family to identify alternative ways in which the hostile interaction could have been handled. Again, throughout all of this, the therapist must carefully confront the problem of the criticisms while not becoming critical him- or herself.

The therapist may find it necessary to call upon the less critical parent to assist in the process of working on these issues. As a resource and ally to the more critical parent, the other parent can often work with his or her partner on ways to decrease critical comments. In other words, try to get the parents to support each other's efforts throughout this difficult process. An overly burdened parent may show exhaustion and frustration by becoming more critical of the patient. Encourage the more energetic and perhaps less critical parent to find ways to support his or her partner in the difficult task of taking on the illness.

What if the therapist becomes exhausted with the parents?

In the same way that the parents may show signs of exhaustion with this process, it is also quite possible for the therapist to become exhausted in the face of little or no progress, especially if he or she has been unable to mobilize the parents, or the therapist feels that he or she has been unable to impress on the parents just how important it is for them to work together as a team. Relatively little can be done to rejuvenate the therapist other than reiterating the fact that, as much as we want this therapy to be a relatively brief affair, AN remains a long-term illness. Both the family's and the therapist's abilities can be severely tested before a turning point in the self-starvation may be reached. It is helpful for the therapist to remain vigilant of his or her own frustrations and to keep these feelings from spilling over into therapy sessions. Regular meetings with a peer could also be helpful in providing the therapist with an opportunity to voice this frustration and to consult with this peer as to how best to proceed with treatment.

What if the patient develops binge eating and purge behaviors?

As has already been noted, the treatment in this manual is appropriate for adolescents with AN. However, some adolescents with AN develop a bingeing-and-purging pattern. Often this happens in the context of weight recovery. Strategies to address this problem within this manualized approach require some comment. Eisler et al. (2000) suggest that with older adolescents who have AN with bulimic symptoms, it is sometimes necessary for the family to acknowledge that they cannot take charge of their daughter's behaviors in this area. They suggest that the therapist might need to capitulate to this finding and focus instead on why the parents still find evidence of her bulimic behaviors if these behaviors are indeed not their concerns. The strategy, then, is not focused on parental management but on how eating behaviors are still a means of communicating within the family. For younger patients, though, there may still be scope within the confines of this manual for parents to address this issue. In some instances, it may be appropriate for parents to extend their vigilance, which until now has concentrated on the prevention of self-starvation, to include the prevention of binge eating and vomiting. The therapist should encourage the patient to eat healthy amounts of food at mealtimes, thereby helping the patient learn once more how much food may be appropriate at any sitting. It is not uncommon to have the parents serve the patient and help them to learn what quantity is appropriate. Some patients would complain that once they start eating again, they do not know when to stop. There is room for parental involvement at this level. At the same time, parents can be creative in finding ways to help the patient remain constructively engaged after mealtimes to prevent purging. Parents may take turns going for a leisurely walk with the patient after mealtimes or sitting down to watch a favorite movie on television or participating in a hobby activity. In more severe instances, parents may have to resort to drastic measures, such as accompanying an adolescent to the bathroom (while waiting outside, of course) in similar fashion to what is done on a specialist inpatient unit. Likewise, parents may have to lock the kitchen cupboards to prevent patients from binge eating. As with the prevention of self-starvation, the aim is not to prescribe for the parents how they should proceed. Rather, the aim is to help the parents understand that this is a serious illness and that they need to find ways that will work for them and their family to prevent their daughter from starving herself or, as in this example, from binge eating and purging.

What if the therapy is not working?

In the psychiatric treatment of AN, perhaps more so than for any other psychiatric disorder, the therapist may find that his or her work is evaluated in a very concrete way through weekly weight recordings that put his or her work with the patient and her family on visual display in the form of a weight chart. The therapist must not respond to the patient's weight loss as though he or she were the one failing in treatment. Such a response may only undermine the therapist's ability to implement this manualized treatment effectively. In such instances, the therapist ought to examine how he or she may have to go about treatment differently to enable the parents to find a solution to their daughter's eating problem. In other words, the question to be examined is what is impeding the parents in their task at refeeding. Although the therapist may feel "on display" when the patient fails to gain weight, our experience with these families indicates that the families are much more likely to feel that they are not succeeding in the task than to blame the therapist for "incompetence." The families' tendency to be self-critical should, of course, not serve to exonerate the therapist from responsibility for creating the "right" treatment environment, one in which the parents are mobilized to take on the difficult task of refeeding their child.

What about suicidal or self-injurious patients?

It is not uncommon for adolescents with AN to become seriously depressed or to demonstrate incipient signs of a personality disorder. The approaches to these two kinds of problems are quite different.

• *Suicidal patients.* Adolescent suicide is a major cause of death among teenagers in the United States. Suicidal behaviors need to be taken seriously and managed as an emergency. It is impossible to continue to focus on the disordered eating problems as a cause of morbidity and potential mortality when a patient is actively suicidal. Only after the acute situation of a suicidal behavior has subsided can the family and patient be expected to continue with family treatment for AN.

• *Self-injurious behaviors.* Self-injurious behavior that is nonlethal and not suicidal in intent can emerge among patients with AN. These behaviors may have always been a part of the patient's presentation, or, more commonly, they may emerge as challenges to the disordered eating behaviors by parents or professionals increase. These types of behaviors may include such things as cutting or scraping parts of the body, rubbing, picking, pulling out hair, pinching, and so forth. None of the behaviors are themselves intended to be life threatening; their aims may be variously described as self-punishing, anxiety relieving, dissociative, or ritualistic. Sometimes these behaviors can escalate to the point at which they become life endangering, but most of the time they are not. They are extremely upsetting for parents and sometimes for therapists as well. We see these types of behaviors as part of an overall communication pattern within the family and, like the disordered eating, a substitute for more effective communication. Thus, as long as these behaviors remain at a moderately low level, we proceed with therapy according to the model described, with a focus on the disordered eating as the behavior mostly likely to cause the greatest harm. These behaviors, if they persist, may become a greater part of the focus in Phase III, in which some of the underlying conflicts may be explored actively after the disordered eating has been set aside. If these behaviors do indeed escalate and become a greater hazard than the disordered eating, they may need to become the focus for treatment for a time.

How does one assess readiness for Phase II?

Careful scrutiny of the parents' performance as a unified team in refeeding their daughter, steady weight gain for the patient, support for the patient's dilemma from the parents, and reinforcement of sibling sympathy and understanding for their sister's struggle are the main focus points throughout Sessions 3 to 10. The first sign of the family's readiness to move to Phase II of treatment may be reduced anxiety and tension in non-food-related discussions. Steady weight gain, however, is the main yardstick by which the therapist assesses the family's readiness to progress to Phase II of treatment. Therefore, treatment will progress to Phase II only when steady weight gain has been established and the parents feel confident in their ability to ensure a healthy weight for their adolescent offspring, in addition to having accomplished the abovementioned tasks. It is possible that many patients will not require the full 10 sessions to complete this phase; others may continue in this phase a good deal longer.

How can the therapist's response to families affect treatment?

We now briefly discuss how the therapist's feelings toward a particular family might affect the treatment approach described in this manual. We take two extremes of response as a way of illustrating the overall problems: liking a family and disliking a family.

• *Liking a family.* It may seem that liking a family is an important element in engaging them in treatment. To a certain extent, this is certainly true. However, if one likes a family too much, specific problems can arise in implementing the therapy described here. In the early sessions in Phase I, holding a family in too positive regard may make it difficult to generate the correct mix of anxiety and trepidation, as well as competence, that the therapist wishes to engender in the family. For example, it may be more difficult for the therapist to state directly and with intensity the problems AN has caused the family. In other words, the therapist may wish to protect the family too much, to make them feel more relaxed. Yet they may then take the illness and the need for action less seriously. This in turn may lead to their failure to take on the eating problems as strongly as they need to. In a sense, then, by liking the family too much, the therapist enters the system that colludes with ignoring the illness and letting it continue unconfronted.

• *Disliking a family.* Disliking a family can also cause problems. The therapist may try to avoid the family and be distant. This makes the family feel abandoned and unsupported in the monumental battle they need to undertake against AN. Such avoidance and distance may resemble strategies that they have themselves employed with their anorexic child, and they may feel that the therapist is modeling this strategy, even if his or her words say the opposite. If the family feels that the therapist is avoiding them or has abandoned them, it is less likely that the family will succeed in finding the necessary resources to fight the illness. When a therapist dislikes a family, there may be a tendency to be more harsh and critical in their engagements. For example, the therapist might communicate the family's attempts to manage the illness as failures but might do so in a way that models an overly critical stance. Of course, such a stance is the opposite of the one the therapy recommends. Actions, though, may speak louder than words. Increasing criticism would be a particularly unwelcome result because, as we have noted previously, such an attitude may lead to poorer outcome.

We have avoided the term "countertransference" in the preceding discussion, though this might indeed be the proper term in some cases. Instead, we emphasize the importance of the therapist's conscious attitude and behavior toward the patient. In part, the manual itself emphasizes the need for a firm but sympathetic and caring stance. When the therapist notices that he or she is having problems maintaining this stance, careful self-evaluation as to why this is occurring should be undertaken and the problem corrected. One of the reasons that we recommend working in a team and in therapeutic pairs is that it is less likely that problems that result from liking or disliking a patient or a family will go unnoticed. The main corrective to these types of problems, in our opinion, is to try to understand the origin of the feelings and then to take action to get things back on track.

9

Session 8 in Action

*T*he following illustrates a session relatively late in Phase I of treatment. As mentioned, sessions are necessarily less ordered than in the initial session, although still clearly structured around a set of goals that are accomplished via a series of specific interventions.

To review, there are three goals for these treatment sessions:

- To keep the family focused on the eating disorder.
- To help the parents take charge of their daughter's eating.
- To mobilize siblings to support the patient.

In order to accomplish these goals, the following interventions will be appropriate to consider during the remainder of treatment for Phase I:

1. Weighing the patient at the beginning of each session.
2. Directing, redirecting, and focusing therapeutic discussion on food and eating behaviors and their management until food, eating, and weight behaviors and concerns are relieved.
3. Discussing, supporting, and helping the parental dyad's efforts at refeeding.
4. Discussing, supporting, and helping the family to evaluate efforts of siblings to help their affected sister.
5. Continuing to modify parental and sibling criticisms.
6. Continuing to distinguish the adolescent patient and her interests from those of AN.
7. Closing all sessions with a recounting of progress.

Clinical Background

This is a session with the same family described in the clinical vignette from Session 1. At this point the family has clearly taken charge of the adolescent's eating and weight, but they continue to improve in accomplishing the refeeding task. The patient has gained weight to a point where she is out of acute danger but has not yet regained menses. As noted previously, the therapeutic interventions are more fluid than in the first two sessions, which were more scripted. Thus the commentary identifies the interplay of the seven interventions described in the preceding section.

Weighing the Patient at the Beginning of Each Session

As always, the patient was weighed by the therapist prior to beginning the family session. In this case the patient reported that it had been a difficult week with her mother at home without her stepfather to help out.

THERAPIST: I notice that the weight chart has not shown any change this week. What's been happening for the last 2 weeks?

SUSAN: Not much.

MOTHER: We've been working very hard actually . . . umm, seemed to have lost a little weight, so we've been working really hard. . . .

SUSAN: I think the scale was wrong, though . . . I think it was, because one time I stood on it and it was higher, the next time I got on it, a few seconds later, when the nurse's assistant came in it was lower, so I think the scale is off. But . . . my mom doesn't believe me (*laughs*).

THERAPIST: Is this at your pediatrician's?

MOTHER: Yeah.

THERAPIST: How off was the scale?

MOTHER: Two pounds.

SUSAN: I don't think so.

MOTHER: Well, it was 1 pound off from . . . where they had been Wednesday . . . at any rate, she had been down a pound and then she came to the eating disorder clinic and it was a pound heavier than what he had found, but when we went back she was 2 pounds less.

THERAPIST: This was last Friday?

MOTHER: Yeah. So it was off at least a pound. I mean it could have been off a pound, but her weight was off 2 pounds so . . . I don't think it was off 2 pounds. I'm not buying that one.

SUSAN: I think it was off (*laughs again*). Well, we can't check it because she threw our scale away so, I can't . . . I can't see how accurate that was.

In the preceding exchange the therapist explores the meaning of the lack of weight progress based on the weight chart. Because the patient has at least maintained her weight according to the weight chart, the therapist is not terribly alarmed and does not place a great deal of emphasis on this point.

THERAPIST: You decided to throw the scale away?

MOTHER: Yeah. . . .

THERAPIST: You and Tom did?

MOTHER: Yeah, well . . . we had put the scale up and I had told Susan that she was getting weighed three times a week and that was more than enough and, umm, then she sort of decided she wanted to weigh herself anyway, so she got the scale out of where it had been put up and weighed herself and so we just threw it away. So now we don't have a scale so now we never know what we weigh (*laughs*). But that's okay. Took away the temptation.

THERAPIST: So this was a mutual decision you and Tom made about this?

MOTHER: Yeah.

THERAPIST: Before we move on . . . where is Tom today? Is he okay?

MOTHER: Yeah. He had to go to out of town for the week and so he was just getting back and there was no way we could have juggled it to get him here in time, so, unfortunately, that's where he's at.

THERAPIST: I see. So, this is kind of the inverse of the week when you were gone . . . any comparisons as to how the week went?

MOTHER: You'd have to compare it with her because I wasn't there the last week (*laughs*).

In the following exchange, the therapist is exploring how a decision was made by Susan's parents about managing Susan's wish to weigh herself and an example of her parents' efforts at refeeding.

Discussing, Supporting, and Helping Parental Dyad's Efforts at Refeeding

In this session, one of the parents is missing, so the therapist wants to understand why. It is notable that this is whole-family therapy, and though one family member is missing, it is possible to continue therapy for one session when there is an urgent reason a parent has to be away, especially at this point in therapy.

SUSAN: I think it went just fine. We're getting along very well, I think. She, umm (*laughs*) . . . Oh my! I found it amusing, I wasn't angry. I mean obviously she's trying to fatten me up but, . . . she was so nice when I came home from school and she was like, "I made you pudding . . . but I made it with fat-free milk so it's gonna taste. . . . "

MOTHER: No, I never . . . I never said that . . . I said I made it . . . I didn't make it with whole milk so it might take longer to set. . . .

SUSAN: She said I didn't make it with whole milk so it's going to take longer to set . . . she made it sound as if she used the fat-free milk . . . in the fridge and . . . unbeknownst to me she had used Boost in it also but I could detect this when I tasted it. I said this tastes suspiciously like chocolate-raspberry Boost . . . she got this guilty little grin on her face (*laughs*) "Well I know you love me so I'm not going to be angry."

THERAPIST: Did it taste good, though?

SUSAN: It tasted okay. It was just . . . it was funny I was, like, well, you know what . . . I'm not going to tell my friends about this because then they'll never eat anything their mothers make for them again.

THERAPIST: (*to mother*) Was that something you thought to do . . . what was your thought process . . . deciding to make the pudding? She says you're trying to fatten her up.

SUSAN: Sneaking calories that I didn't think were there.

MOTHER: Well, actually I wasn't trying to be . . . uh, I wasn't necessarily trying to be deceptive because I don't think that's good because she needs to be able to trust me. So that's why when she asked me . . . I said I made you pudding, but I didn't use whole milk . . . I let her kind of assume . . . But my thought process was the Boost. She's been having a hard time getting proteins and things and I've been encouraging her to drink three cans of Boost everyday.

THERAPIST: That's great . . .

MOTHER: But she doesn't really like to do it. And a long time ago we had talked about Boost pudding and so I got to thinking about, well, maybe if I just put the Boost in the pudding that will give her a better source of protein, so that's why I initially did it. I figured she'd be able to taste it because you know it's pretty hard to get around that.

THERAPIST: So your thought was she likes pudding . . . and you had a joking conversation about Boost pudding? . . .

MOTHER: When she was in the hospital we used to talk about, "Well, they oughta make Boost pudding and Boost cake" because, you know . . . the "no Boost" thing, and so I was always saying they oughta have all these other things, so I thought I would just add it, and I wasn't even sure it would set in the pudding or not but. . . .

SUSAN: And it didn't really.

MOTHER: It just sort of. . . .

SUSAN: It was runny.

MOTHER: It's a little soft, it's kind of like what if would have been if you made it strictly with skim milk.

THERAPIST: It's sounds like it was a really creative idea and also it sounds to me like it was fun too. (*to Susan*) You even kind of enjoyed it, sounds like.

SUSAN: I thought it was kind of funny . . . I'm like yeah, I can just imagine now, she's like, "I'll scramble you an egg, Susan." And she's probably like throwing in like lard and stuff trying to sneak in extra calories (*laughs*). I think I'll scramble my own eggs from now on.

MOTHER: I've never put anything in your scrambled eggs.

SUSAN: Well, how do I know (*laughs*)?

THERAPIST: Is your mom making more stuff for you now . . . because didn't you used to make more of your own meals?

SUSAN: Umm, yeah, and I think I still do make some. . . .

MOTHER: It kind of depends on what we're having and what she feels like having . . . like last night I made soup and we kind of just added to it. . . .

SUSAN: It was supposed to be potato soup and it was more like. . . .

THERAPIST: It was like stone soup?

MOTHER: Yeah, it just sort of got everything thrown into it . . . it was pretty good though.

THERAPIST: You don't agree, Paul?

MOTHER: He doesn't like potato soup so. . . . (*laughs*) and he really dislikes vegetables and it had all kinds of stuff in it.

THERAPIST: Did you guys try the pudding?

MOTHER: They didn't know it even had Boost in it so. . . .

PAUL: I didn't even know you made pudding!

THERAPIST: Would you have liked to try it?

MOTHER AND SUSAN: It's still there (*laughter*).

SUSAN: An awful lot of it.

Directing, Redirecting, and Focusing the Therapeutic Discussion on Food and Eating Behaviors and Their Management until Food, Eating, and Weight Behaviors and Concerns Are Relieved

THERAPIST: So, are there other creative things you've tried throughout the week . . . that's one example that. . . .

MOTHER: Well, we shared lunch today . . . we went out and we ordered chicken parmesan and we shared that . . . that was kind of fun and we've been trying to be inventive and get things that she likes to eat so that we can get the calories down.

SUSAN: We have a lot of crackers and ice cream in our house.

MOTHER: If we run out we just get more.

THERAPIST: You mean those go together?

MOTHER: No, the crackers go with the jelly . . . or with the cream cheese. Then the . . . it's not exactly ice cream. . . .

SUSAN: I've probably eaten like . . . almost two boxes of ice cream in the last couple of days.

THERAPIST: That's a lot of ice cream.

SUSAN: Well, one of them was frozen yogurt.

PAUL: I don't like the frozen yogurt stuff . . . that stuff is sick.

SUSAN: You never tried it!

PAUL: Yes, I did.

SUSAN: The chocolate peanut butter cup?

THERAPIST: You like to stick to ice cream? It's not no calorie, it's "light."

MOTHER: It's "light," yeah.

SUSAN: But I could get the other one if I wanted to. . . .

MOTHER: It has the same amount of calories as frozen yogurt, basically, so . . . and it doesn't have any fat.

THERAPIST: Okay. So, what was it like having lunch together? Sharing lunch . . . that sounds like a nice plan.

SUSAN: It was okay. The boys were at school we were about to go pick them up and so . . . I had just gotten out of school and we thought, "Let's go get some lunch" . . . so we went out . . . that was fun.

THERAPIST: You went out to a restaurant?

SUSAN: Normally my boyfriend and I order that, umm . . . it's his favorite thing so he's like "it's really good, you have to try it." And the chicken is like one big piece so I don't have to eat it, I just try a little.

MOTHER: We were attempting to try a little bit of chicken . . . I mean, microscopically, but we got a little, tiny, weenie piece of chicken in.

THERAPIST: How'd you do that?

MOTHER: Well, I asked her if she'd like to try it and so she tried a little, tiny piece.

THERAPIST: Sounds like you were worried about the proteins. . . .

MOTHER: Yeah. Yeah, she's really not getting a lot of protein . . . she eats a lot of vegetables and she's been *eating* but she's not getting the food that has really primarily a lot of protein so I keep trying to get her more protein.

PAUL: Kind of bad like if you don't like beans or anything (*laughs*).

SUSAN: I like beans . . . I eat plenty of them.

PAUL: You used to hate beans!

SUSAN: I don't want pork and beans.

THERAPIST: You know that's a good protein source (*to Paul*) . . . beans and rice.

MOTHER: Yeah, well, we don't do the rice either, so . . . (*pointedly at Susan*).

SUSAN: I do rice.

MOTHER: Not in a blue moon. You haven't had any rice for a while, for quite a while.

SUSAN: Well, maybe I just haven't felt like it. . . . I'm not trying to . . . what's in rice?

MOTHER: I don't know.

SUSAN: Not much.

In the preceding exchanges, the therapist keeps the focus on food and weight concerns and actively explores and supports the parents' efforts at refeeding. In this case, there are a number of important examples of efforts, some of which worked better than others. For example, the pudding was a mixed success, probably in part because there was a level of deception that undermined the effort. On the other hand, making sure there are foods that are acceptable and nutritious seemed effective, as well as supportively taking Susan out to a restaurant. The therapist is never critical of the parents' efforts and looks for positive statements to make about their efforts.

THERAPIST: The beans and the rice are complementary in terms of the amino acids you need, so that would be a nice thing you might consider. If it's microscopic it's still progress, but. . . .

MOTHER: We're working on it . . . we're trying to increase her eggs . . . she doesn't like eggs but we're working on it.

THERAPIST: Now, during this week . . . when you were away you checked in with Tom regularly. He'll check in with you, and you guys are on the same page, as it were, about what you're doing?

MOTHER: Yeah.

THERAPIST: Good.

MOTHER: We worked out a point system that Susan's excited about. I hope that will be beneficial.

THERAPIST: What's that?

SUSAN: Umm, every time I go to clinic on Friday and maintain my weight I get 100 dollars, every time I go and I gain weight I get 200 and when I reach 130, I get 1,000, and it goes into an account for a new car.

THERAPIST: Wow.

SUSAN: Yeah!

THERAPIST: How much money has she collected?

SUSAN: None yet because they canceled clinic today!

MOTHER: Well, we haven't really started because they canceled clinic today after all that . . . they canceled the eating disorder clinic today.

SUSAN: So, I can't prove that that scale is wrong and so no one believes me, but I know that it is. Because there's no way that I couldn't have gained with all I've been eating . . . no way.

THERAPIST: Let me ask you, is this above the last highest weight that she has to gain?

MOTHER: Above where she was, yes.

THERAPIST: Because you could lose weight and then gain. . . .

MOTHER: No . . . if she loses she doesn't lose any money, but she doesn't get anything at all.

THERAPIST: You understand what I'm saying, though. . . .

MOTHER: Yes, she has to keep gaining. . . .

THERAPIST: She was at 100 and she lost at 95 and the next week she went to 97 . . . she gained but she didn't gain above 100.

SUSAN: Oh no, I don't know. We didn't talk about that.

MOTHER: Well, she shouldn't get anything if she loses until she gets back up to where she was before she quit. And also the other thing that her Dad and I have discussed, but we haven't really discussed with her . . . was self-injury . . . that is, she has self-injury, she loses 100 bucks. She doesn't know about that. . . .

SUSAN: We didn't talk about that (*some laughter*).

MOTHER: She doesn't know about that part, but that . . . that's kind of important, because especially when she gains sometimes it's hard for her, and she tends to injure herself, as you all know.

The therapist explores how the parents are going to implement a point system that they have devised to motivate Susan. The therapist carefully points out some possible pitfalls but does not criticize the approach.

THERAPIST: Umm, that sounds like a good plan, too. So this is motivating . . . yet it's hard to know whether it's working.

MOTHER: Yeah, it's too soon to know yet, but. . . .

THERAPIST: You guys have done a lot of things.

MOTHER: We're trying to be creative . . . we'll try just about anything.

THERAPIST: Let's see now, you've come up with . . . Boost pudding, sharing a meal, and this point system. Now one of the other things that had been going on was that Susan had not been eating with you at dinner, and that was corrected then several weeks ago. But I was wondering if it's still continuing.

MOTHER: Pretty much so . . . sometimes she has a hard time waiting until we actually eat, so if that happens and she wants to eat before we actually sit down to eat, then she'll normally sit down and eat something with us at that point in time, so . . . pretty much we try to. . . . She pretty much comes out, and she's not like in the beginning, she would take her food into her room and she didn't want anyone to see her eating at all, and we've kind of gotten past that . . . pretty much, huh? She pretty much eats everything, umm. . . .

SUSAN: That's for sure. I eat everything! I'm surprised we have food in our house still as much as I eat! I'm serious!

MOTHER: She eats a lot but she measures everything. So, for her a lot is like . . . and I kind of get after her . . . like yesterday she was fixing chili for lunch and she had a half a cup, and I told her a half a cup just wasn't enough. So. . . .

SUSAN: But I was having other stuff!

MOTHER: She added some other things to it, but I'm going to be really happy when she quits feeling the need to measure everything, where she can just put portions on her plate and eat it and not worry about how many calories there are. . . . We haven't quite gotten there yet.

THERAPIST: So are you and Tom feeling like you have to still be closely monitoring her?

MOTHER: Yes.

SUSAN: I don't think so . . . because I eat. . . .

MOTHER: You've never thought so. . . .

SUSAN: No, but really . . . I eat when they're not around, like when she's asleep, I go into the kitchen and I eat . . . I eat until the time I go to sleep, and I'm normally up pretty late, and I'll like be eating at 12 o'clock in the morning.

PAUL: Yeah, I've heard her eating chips in her bedroom at 12 o'clock in the night. . . .

MOTHER: But she only eats like six chips. . . .

SUSAN: That's not true. . . .

MOTHER: Usually when you eat them you eat very small amounts, and you tend to put them in little baggies, and when you're out of the baggy, you tend to not eat any more.

SUSAN: That's not true . . . I, like, polished off a whole bag of crackers last night . . . all by myself.

MOTHER: Well, the crackers are kind of a new thing. We go through fads, and crackers are kind of the new thing.

THERAPIST: Crackers with jelly?

MOTHER: Uh, no, sometimes just plain . . . sometimes with cream cheese . . . it just kind of depends.

THERAPIST: But you like cream cheese?

MOTHER: Oh no, we don't do *regular* cream cheese, but we're doing light . . . 'cause fat free really tastes bad.

SUSAN: No, it doesn't . . . I like strawberry.

MOTHER: Well, the strawberry . . . but the plain really tastes nasty. So that's good! I wish they made it all taste nasty so that she'd have to eat "light" (*laughs*).

SUSAN:: Then I just wouldn't eat it.

The therapist summarizes the efforts at refeeding that the family attempted over the past week then moves on to allow more exploration of how this affects the relationship between Susan and her parents, particularly her mother.

Continuing to Modify Parental and Sibling Criticisms

The therapist notes that the mother struggles with being critical of her daughter, usually using sarcastic humor or minimizing her efforts. In the following exchange, the therapist aims to respect the mother's authority while attempting to modulate her criticism of her daughter. In this regard he hopes to model for her another way of acknowledging Susan's efforts.

THERAPIST: Are you concerned about the amount of fat that she's getting in her diet?

MOTHER: I. . . .

SUSAN: I wouldn't be.

MOTHER: I don't think she gets nearly enough fat in her diet . . . so I am concerned about that. She eats a lot, but she's not necessarily eating all the things that she needs and not in combination . . . yes, she's probably okay calorie-wise . . . a lot of times she's taking in calories, but they're not, you know . . . a Kit Kat bar is not what I would consider *good* nutrition . . . It's calories but it's not really . . . and it's okay . . . so that's like bonus stuff . . . if you want to eat that, that's bonus, but you still have to have the main nutrition and we're . . . we're working on that one. We haven't gotten that one down yet . . . she's still. . . . She really has a hard time with that. . . .

THERAPIST: Well, it's trying . . .

SUSAN: Not really.

MOTHER: Not really?

SUSAN: I'm eating "light" ice cream. . . .

MOTHER: Yes, you're eating "light" ice cream. . . .

SUSAN: And the crackers. . . .

MOTHER: And the crackers are "50%" which is better than we've done . . . so that is an improvement.

THERAPIST: That's terrific.

MOTHER: Yeah.

THERAPIST: But as long as you're still concerned, you might look at some other windows of opportunity . . . What occurred to me as you were talking was that if she likes the cream cheese part . . . that would be a good thing to think about, I don't know how much fat is in cream cheese, but I'm sure there's more in regular cream cheese than in low fat. . . .

SUSAN: There's like 95 calories in regular cream cheese.

THERAPIST: And how many in low fat?

SUSAN: Umm, 25 . . . maybe.

THERAPIST: So that would be an opportunity to add some fat grams, if you're concerned.

MOTHER: The trick is she won't take it, that's the problem.

SUSAN: I'm getting plenty!

THERAPIST: Any other thoughts as to how she might get it? That was just since she likes the crackers and cream cheese. . . .

SUSAN: And all that ice cream . . . 35 grams of . . . I mean 35 fat calories.

It's only like 4 grams of fat in, like, each half a cup, and I go through more than half a cup a day, so I'm sure I'm getting plenty, in spite of what my mother says. I'll . . . she'll never be satisfied with as much as I'm eating, I don't think (*laughs*). She won't be satisfied until I'm like. . . .

MOTHER: No, that's not true. The goal here was never to make you fat. Never has been . . . even though in your mind you think you're fat, that was never the goal. The goal is to make you healthy.

THERAPIST: What will be your and Tom's criterion that you will have for her to be healthy . . . enough so you can be less worried about that.

MOTHER: Well, I think that when she's . . . in our eyes she needs to gain some more weight. She's still under where she needs to be.

THERAPIST: About how much more, do you think?

SUSAN: Barely any. Like 2 pounds.

MOTHER: (*gestures disagreement*).

SUSAN: No, really!

MOTHER: Actually, she used to weigh . . . at one point in time she weighed 140 pounds, and I thought she was light then, but I was willing to accept that because she was able to. . . .

THERAPIST: She was having regular menstrual periods?

MOTHER: Yeah, everything was pretty normal then, although I was concerned at that point in time that she wasn't getting enough protein in her diet also . . . but she was actually maintaining, she had a good energy level, things were pretty much normal at that weight.

SUSAN: I feel good now, though. . . .

MOTHER: And I felt comfortable with, you know . . . I would have liked her to weigh a little bit more but she was, you know, she didn't necessarily *have* to. So, if she could get back up to there. . . .

SUSAN: (*laughter*).

MOTHER: If she could get back up to there, I'd be thrilled . . . (*laughter*) It's gonna be a struggle, I'm sure! Umm, also, if she could just eat regular meals and not have to worry about, you know, looking at everything she eats to see how many calories, how much fat, how much whatever's in the box or whatever she's eating, because nothing goes into her mouth until she's read every nutritional thing on the side of it. . . .

SUSAN: (*softly*) Not true.

MOTHER: I would like to get her past that.

SUSAN: I don't know what was in that chicken parmesan.

MOTHER: Yeah, but you have a pretty good idea. Umm. . . .

THERAPIST: But you didn't eat the chicken part.

SUSAN: No, but I had all that fresh parmesan cheese on the top with the sauce!

THERAPIST: So, the reason I mention that to you is that the criterion that I would be looking for is regular menstrual cycles without any kind of hormonal replacement and between 18 and 25% body fat.

SUSAN: *(laughs)* I'm probably there already . . . I'm probably like 40% *(laughs)*!!

In the preceding series of exchanges, the therapist keeps the focus on eating and healthy weight gain and reinforces the idea that this is about the body's natural healthy weight as determined by menses in women. He attempts to shift the discussion away from calories and weight targets per se to healthy eating and healthy bodies instead.

Continuing to Distinguish the Adolescent Patient and Her Interests from Those of AN

MOTHER: No, you only feel like you are . . . that's that alien in there that thinks that . . . it's not the real person.

SUSAN: It's okay though, because I'm dealing with it, so. . . .

MOTHER: You are . . . you're working on it very hard.

THERAPIST: You made a nice distinction there between Susan and the Alien. It does feel as if Susan's in the room a lot to me.

MOTHER: Yeah, she's here more. You can tell a difference when she's here . . . when the Alien comes to visit, it doesn't have as much power as it used to . . . I've noticed that. Even when it is coming around, she's handling it better. She did have a struggle . . . was it last week . . . that you burned yourself?

SUSAN: It was probably a couple weeks, yeah *(softer)*.

MOTHER: No, it was last week.

SUSAN: No, it wasn't.

MOTHER: Well, you still had the . . . you still had the-they were still very visible last week. Umm, anyway . . . you can tell when he comes out to play . . . I say it's a "he" because you know a woman would never do that, so it's got to be a "he" . . . (*gestures playfully with Paul, to her left*). But it's . . . she is working much harder.

In the preceding exchange, the therapist notes that the "Alien," which is how Susan and the family characterize AN, is more removed from her behaviors both at home and in session. This is continuing to support the clear delineation between AN and Susan herself.

THERAPIST: And you guys are working much harder. I mean it sounds like as parents you're on this pretty . . . do you feel it? Susan, do you feel it . . . that they're really interested in trying to help you?

SUSAN: Yeah.

THERAPIST: Not that you weren't before, but it sounds like you've figured out all lots of active ways to do this.

MOTHER: Well, it's become a way of life. Umm. . . .

THERAPIST: Good . . . good.

MOTHER: We, ugh . . . we had a little bit of a setback . . . Elizabeth came last week . . . was it last week . . . ?

THERAPIST: Elizabeth?

MOTHER: Elizabeth is a friend that was hospitalized the same time that Susan was, and she came home for the weekend.

THERAPIST: Does she have an eating disorder?

MOTHER: Yeah.

THERAPIST: Did you guys meet her (*to the two brothers*)?

PAUL: Yeah, we've known her for a *long* time.

THERAPIST: You knew her from. . . .

MOTHER: The hospital . . . yeah.

THERAPIST: So you know who she. . . .

MOTHER: She's a *very* nice young lady, but she's having a very hard time right now with her eating disorder . . . and it was very hard. I could see Susan having a hard time, and she may not have noticed it, but watching her try to deal with . . . you know, she was trying to encourage Elizabeth to eat and she wasn't really into eating, and then Susan would kind of pull back, and I noticed that by the time the weekend was over I was very concerned, because Susan had decreased the amount she was eating down to where she would have a half a cup of vegetables, and that was what she ate

... she was full, and I was like, "wait a minute, we're going backwards here," and it's taken us about a week to get kind of back. . . .

THERAPIST: Did you talk to Susan about your concerns?

MOTHER: I talked to Susan about it when Elizabeth was at the house and told her that I was very concerned about her but also that I was very concerned about Elizabeth, because she wasn't eating, either.

THERAPIST: Did you guys notice that, too?

SUSAN: I was eating.

MOTHER: Well, you'd come out and eat some when Elizabeth wasn't there, but it was still a bit of a struggle for you, I can see it.

SUSAN: It really wasn't, and I hate that . . . how everyone always thinks it's so bloody hard and it's not always so hard, you know. I can eat and I'm not always. . . .

MOTHER: Well, you did cut down your amounts substantially. . . .

SUSAN: I don't think so. I really don't think so.

THERAPIST: So you noticed an influence of a peer . . . what you felt was an influence, and you don't agree with that (*to Susan*), but you did notice it, and so you tried to address it. There is a really powerful culture around diet and food and weight among adolescent girls, right? You would agree, right?

SUSAN: (*nods*).

THERAPIST: And it's particularly powerful in subcultures, including eating disorders . . . so even if it wasn't so, it's good to be alert to it. It sounds like you were pretty confident with what you saw, but the reality is, it's powerful.

MOTHER: Yeah, it was very powerful. Even Susan, when she was in the hospital, noticed that some of the girls that weren't in the hospital with an eating disorder tended to start having some problems with that just by being around the girls that were . . . we talked about that. . . .

THERAPIST: You noticed that (*gesturing to Susan*)?

SUSAN: (*nods*).

MOTHER: And she would encourage them to eat . . . and say you're not like us, you need to eat (*laughs slightly*).

SUSAN: No (*laughter*) "You don't want to be like us."

MOTHER: And she encourages Elizabeth . . . they talk back and forth on the phone, and she's really been encouraging Elizabeth to eat . . . I don't know whether it's working but . . . Those demands are coming out hard and strong, huh?

THERAPIST: Does that same voice encourage you to eat?

SUSAN: Well . . . I don't think that I am having such a hard time. I think I'm doing very well. I, umm. . . .

MOTHER: I would believe that if the scale didn't keep going down . . . (laughter).

SUSAN: Well, that's not my fault, I swear that scale has to be wrong . . . there's no way. It's not possible that I'm eating that much and not gaining weight. It's just not. I'm certain it's wrong.

THERAPIST: What will happen if you get to the scale and it isn't wrong?

SUSAN: What do you mean . . . I have lost?

THERAPIST: (nods).

SUSAN: Well, then, that's just a weird fluke, because it's not possible to eat as much as I've been eating and not gain or at least maintain.

MOTHER: It is if you eat food that has no calories . . . a lot of times you do like a salad and basically your salad has lettuce and carrots and fat-free dressing, which has 15 calories. That's nothing. It's a filler. And sugar-free Kool-Aid is a filler.

SUSAN: That's not all I eat, though.

MOTHER: So . . . they don't all count.

SUSAN: They do count! (smiling)

MOTHER: She has this weird way of counting calories too, that it was funny but . . . and I could see a difference in Susan. because she had gotten this Kit Kat bar. She had decided that she wanted this Kit Kat bar and she told me that she wasn't going to eat as much for dinner because she was having to eat this Kit Kat bar . . . so I just as well know . . . that she was having this (laughter from Susan). So she was sitting there and she's eating this Kit Kat bar but she's taking all the chocolate off of it. She biting all the chocolate off of it and spitting it into her cup because she's not going to eat that. So I said "Yeah! You're going to count this as all of your calories, but you're not eating all of your calories . . . you're spitting them into the cup!" And she goes, "Well . . . " and then she said, "Chocolate does have a lot of calories . . . "

SUSAN: I wasn't counting . . . I wasn't counting it for like 400 calories, which it was though. So. . . .

MOTHER: It was kind of funny. . . .

THERAPIST: But you didn't get into a battle about the number of calories (*to mother*).

MOTHER: No.

THERAPIST: That was good.

MOTHER: . . . and that was the good thing. And the other good thing was that she didn't . . . it used to be that if I'd say, "Susan, you need to eat more," she'd really bounce back on me, "No, I don't! Leave me alone!" And now I'll say, "Susan, I would really like it if you'd eat that apple." She'll look at me and say, "You'd really like it if I eat that apple?" (*laughter*) I'll go . . . "Yeah, I'd really like it." Then she'll eat it or she'll eat part of it, which is *good*. So, we're not battling quite so much over food anymore.

THERAPIST: And what have you and Tom done that's made the difference?

MOTHER: I don't . . .

THERAPIST: Because it has changed . . . you've done something

MOTHER: We just keep hammering away . . . and she's making a lot of progress herself. You can't say that we've done everything, but she's certainly put a lot of effort into it.

THERAPIST: You've been persistent.

MOTHER: Well, you know, I'm like the shadow when I'm at home.

THERAPIST: Well that's something you did that's been really important . . . you're really there all the time.

MOTHER: Yeah . . . we're there (*laughter*).

THERAPIST: What about school . . . are you eating at school?

SUSAN: Umm, normally.

MOTHER: Actually, she eats before she goes to school, and then she takes something to snack on usually at school, and then I pick her up at lunchtime. So she's not at school during meals. She eats before she goes, and then like yesterday she took a Boost bar with her, and then I pick her up if she's going . . . she only goes Mondays, Wednesdays, Fridays in the morning, and so she eats before she goes, and then she eats when she gets home at lunch. And then on Tuesdays and Thursdays she goes in the afternoon, so she's eaten breakfast and lunch before she goes to school and she eats again later so we really don't have . . . she's really not at school during mealtimes.

THERAPIST: So you've been able to keep an eye on that.

MOTHER: Yeah, pretty much.

THERAPIST: When we met last time, umm, one of the things that came up was that Susan had done well for one of the weeks and not as well the second week, and . . . one of the differences was she'd gone back to school, and I wondered if you thought that going . . . and that was when we weren't sure what that meant.

MOTHER: Well, I'm not sure . . . I didn't think it was, when she went to school I didn't think it was because she wasn't eating because she was at school. I felt more that it might be because of the stress of going to school. . . .

SUSAN: I'm . . . I'm . . . I'm actually pretty happy where I'm at right now. I feel pretty good so I'm not . . . I'm not trying to lose weight right now, and if I am it's really by no means of my own because I'm not purging and I'm eating an awful lot.

THERAPIST: That's terrific . . . she's still not purging (*toward mother*).

MOTHER: No.

THERAPIST: That's been how long now?

MOTHER: Three weeks?

SUSAN: I'm not sure.

MOTHER: I think it's 3 weeks this week.

THERAPIST: Well, you hadn't purged till maybe 2 weeks ago. . . .

MOTHER: Yeah, so it's 3 weeks today.

THERAPIST: That's terrific. That's terrific.

THERAPIST: How did you do that?

MOTHER: She quit eating. The anorexic part took over.

THERAPIST: Well, that's what happens at the beginning.

MOTHER: And then that . . . but then she's been increasing her eating, but so far . . . and we do inventive things sometimes, too, because after she eats we go and do things . . . and it's certainly not . . . it's not quite as . . . I wouldn't say it's not as easy, it was just, she could sit there right beside me and purge if she wanted to . . . she's really good at it . . . umm, but. . . .

Discussing, Supporting, and Helping the Family to Evaluate Efforts of Siblings to Help Their Affected Sister

THERAPIST: So you've been doing things to distract her afterward (*to the two brothers*). . . .

PAUL: Yeah. . . .

SUSAN: Well . . . I don't need to be distracted, though, because I . . . the temptation's really not there. I'm . . . it's just not (*pause*). No one's distracting me when I eat on my own or when I eat with my friends and I don't purge then. . . .

MOTHER: But you don't normally eat your meals with your friends.

SUSAN: But I do.

MOTHER: Not normally.

SUSAN: Well, normally no one's home when I'm home. If Connie or Jenny comes over, then they're the only ones who would be around, but still. . . .

THERAPIST: Paul, have you done anything to support your sister this week?

PAUL: Uh, well, I don't know. I guess I talked to her a lot.

SUSAN: Yeah, that was nice.

THERAPIST: How about you, Dan? Anything you can think of?

DAN: I guess I talked to her, too. I didn't try the Boost pudding.

SUSAN: Oh, well, that would be support.

THERAPIST: Anything else?

DAN: I can't think of anything.

THERAPIST: How about you Susan? Can you think of anything they did?

SUSAN: Well, Paul was really nice to me all week. That was great. Dan was, too. That always helps.

In this family, the younger brothers are particularly close to their sister, who in some ways takes care of them like a mother. Although they are quiet in this and many of the sessions, it is clear that their mere presence helps bolster Susan at times. They are regularly supportive of her as a person, and the fact that they are unable to find much in specific that they did to help this week does not alarm the therapist because there is also no criticism of her from them that needs to be modified. Nonetheless, the therapist wants to continue to have them involved in the session and to support their efforts.

THERAPIST: But that's a change then because before I remember . . . the last session that we had together, which would be about 4 weeks ago . . . you were saying that you were having a tough time with temptation . . . this urge after meals. And then you were thinking about ways to distract her after meals. But what you've observed I think is really an accurate pattern, which is . . . the way she got around that was to restrict calories, and then she didn't feel the urge as much. It sounds like now you're working toward getting the calories up. You are very pleased with the progress. You know it's not there . . . you feel it is there (*to Susan*), but the scales will tell us.

MOTHER: Even if it's only a little gain.

THERAPIST: I'm just remembering being a teenager. If she gains a little, it's $200 . . . for 5 weeks, you're going to get a lot of money pretty quick there. Is there any kind of standard . . . (*laughter*).

MOTHER: We figured out that if she were to consistently gain, stay the same or gain, she would accumulate about $500 by the middle of August, which hopefully by that time will have given her enough time to have gotten kind of into eating normally and, uh, not feeling so bad about gaining. And that's about the time then we could be out and start looking for a car . . . but then if she gets what she wants and then she starts losing weight again the keys go away (*laughter*). So you know . . . there's always consequences to her actions.

THERAPIST: You and Tom thought it out . . . so you're not concerned if the weight gains are small. . . .

MOTHER: No.

THERAPIST: . . . as long as they're in the right direction.

MOTHER: I hope so, but I'm not going to count my chickens.

THERAPIST: So . . . the point is as long as she remains below 90 to 95% [of ideal body weight] all the chronic malnutrition issues are not being resolved . . . umm, will continue . . . bone problems, cardiac problems, menstrual problems, et cetera. So, although I think we're going in the right direction, there may need to be a little bit of pressure to help her go a little faster.

SUSAN: I think I'm going fast enough . . . I don't have very far to go.

THERAPIST: Actually, while you're going this way ... (*motions up and down*).

SUSAN: I'm not though ... I'm going. ...

MOTHER: This way (*motions down*).

SUSAN: Up ... and I don't have very much higher to go.

MOTHER: We're supposed to have gone this way (*motions up*).

SUSAN: I just have a couple more pounds before I'm at my, umm. ...

MOTHER: Well, no, that's what your mind is telling you, but that's not what the scale is saying. ...

SUSAN: That's what the target is!

MOTHER: But your mind is saying you only have a couple more pounds but that in reality isn't true, because the scale said 125 and the target was 130. That's 5 pounds.

THERAPIST: Who decided on the target?

MOTHER: Well, I don't know, because that's really low.

SUSAN: That's not low! Give me a break!

MOTHER: I'm not sure how the nutritionist determined 130 because 130. ...

SUSAN: That's not low!

MOTHER: ... for her height and body build. ...

SUSAN: It's not ... it's not low.

THERAPIST: Yeah, I'm just not certain where the 130 came from.

SUSAN: I swear it came from the nutritionist. I'm not just making up numbers.

MOTHER: Well, unfortunately, because at the eating disorder clinic the parents ... and I guess it's probably my biggest complaint about the whole thing is that I feel like I'm the quarterback ... I've been given, you know it's like I've been given this ball and been told to make the touchdown, but I don't have any help. Nobody else on the team knows, you know ... it's like ... when she's in the hospital, everybody knows what we're doing, all that kind of stuff ... not ... not parents, but everybody else knows everything that's going on. But the parents know nothing. Then she's discharged and the same thing continues. We're not even allowed to know how much she weighs unless she tells us how much she weighs. I have no way of knowing how much she weighs, what ... I never get to talk to the nutritionist ... you always get kicked out of the room. So there's no . . . there's no conversation with the nutrition-ist, with Susan, to determine what her . . . what she really needs to be doing and what we can work on. It's very frustrating because it's like you're given all the responsibility to help your child and of course you want to help your child, but you're given none of the information to do it with. . . .

THERAPIST: . . . We will tell you the weights, when we do them here.

MOTHER: But it's . . . it's very frustrating, it's like how much body fat? How do I know? I'm not allowed to know that. Umm, you know. Then they ask you, "do you have any questions," in the eating dis-order clinic, and you say, "Oh yeah, well I wanted to know . . . " and they just kind of skirt the issue and you never really find out anything. It's kind of useless. Last time when she asked us if we had any questions, I said, "Nope . . . don't have any." She said, "You don't have any?" It's like . . . well, you're not going to tell me anything anyway! So . . . what good does it do?

THERAPIST: So, well, we'll try . . . what we can give you here is her prog-ress from session to session. And it sounds like you do know the weight . . . somehow. . . .

MOTHER: Well, Susan has told me. . . .

THERAPIST: You saw the scale?

MOTHER: No . . . no, she told me the last time. And we've been talking. We tried to discuss it, as far as how her vital signs are, how her rate is and things like that. So, umm, she's gotten better with tell-ing me that. Initially, when we first started this she never told me. So it's better.

THERAPIST: Well, it's seems like the points or the money you're getting is based on the weights at the clinic? . . . So you need to have a way to confirm that.

MOTHER: (nods).

THERAPIST: So, Susan, you can tell them that they can share that infor-mation with your mother. Otherwise, you'll never get $200.

THERAPIST: No, they know that. I'm not going to lie to them. I mean, if I was going to lie I wouldn't have told her that the scale said 125.

THERAPIST: So do you feel like . . . Do you (to mother) feel like you could go that route, or do you need to have the confirmation with the clinic?

MOTHER: Well, I think that . . . you know . . . I . . . I would like to have the confirmation with the clinic. Not because I don't trust her, but

I know that, I know that . . . I know that the eating disorder sometimes likes to . . . you know, "Well, I like staying the same . . . "
Okay. You're the same. Well, then you find out, whoops, no,
you're not the same, you lost 2 pounds. So . . . sometimes . . . because in her mind it's the same, but it's not really the same because she doesn't see it that way.

THERAPIST: So for this. . . .

SUSAN: Normally people's weights vary, you know.

MOTHER: Well, they might go up or they might go down, but they don't
always go down.

SUSAN: Well, when it's so exact and . . . people vary and if I had eaten
more that day than I normally did or. . . .

THERAPIST: Yeah, but their $200 is riding on it (*gesturing to mother*). So
let's see now, it sounds like you need for Susan to give them permission.

Again, the preceding series of exchanges is a good example of the therapist's continued exploration of weight and eating concerns and their
management. He keeps the family focused on this, and though there is
again a return to discussion of target weights and calories, the struggle
is short, and it is clear that Susan has capitulated to her parents' demands that she eat.

SUSAN: She doesn't need it . . . we didn't discuss that before and I'm not
going to lie to you and I don't think that they should have to tell
you.

MOTHER: Well . . . but if I don't . . . we did agree that we would go by
the clinic weight . . . we didn't. . . .

SUSAN: We did and you said if you lied to us there wouldn't be anything.

THERAPIST: How would they know if you lied?

SUSAN: They just have to trust me . . . somewhere along the line I have
to have a little trust. I mean . . . "hello." I can't be baby-sat my
whole life.

THERAPIST: Maybe after a certain point that would be a reasonable
thing.

SUSAN: I think I reached that point . . . how long have I been out of the
hospital now?

MOTHER: Five weeks and losing.

SUSAN: No, I'm not.

MOTHER: Well, the trick is you are. You are losing . . . you have maintained 5 weeks, which is wonderful, and every single day out of the hospital is good. The trick is that . . . if your weight continues to go down you're not going to stay out of the hospital.

SUSAN: It's not going down. I'm telling you it is so wrong you don't even know (*smiling*) . . . that scale is wrong. I am certain.

MOTHER: It's consistently wrong.

THERAPIST: When's your next appointment?

MOTHER: Well, the pediatrician is on Monday.

THERAPIST: Maybe you should base them on the pediatrician's . . .

MOTHER: But their scale is. . . .

SUSAN: Their scales are wacko. . . .

MOTHER: Their scale is not as accurate.

SUSAN: It's never on zero when I stand on it.

THERAPIST: But you don't have that information.

MOTHER: But. . . .

SUSAN: But they . . . I haven't ever lied about it before?

MOTHER: Well . . . not exactly lied. You have said it stayed the same when it actually kind of went down. We . . . we found out that you were 2 pounds lighter, uh, than what we had thought you were.

SUSAN: Well, it stayed the same compared to what . . . you didn't ask from what visit had it varied.

MOTHER: (*exasperated sigh*).

The therapist tries to ascertain the level of independence that Susan has over her eating and the level of trust that needs to be present before her parents can allow her more independent eating. It appears to the therapist that the parents are mindful of their daughter's progress but correctly concerned that she has not progressed enough. The therapist remains alert to the underlying but consistently present criticism from Susan's mother and tries to intervene to modify this behavior.

THERAPIST: You're laughing, aren't you? How come you're laughing? (*to Dan*)

DAN: Stayed the same . . . like 3 weeks ago that's what it was at (*laughter*).

THERAPIST: Kind of slippery . . . I see . . . I see.

MOTHER: Do you think you'd get away with that? Do you think I'd let you get away with that?

SUSAN: I don't know.

THERAPIST: Sounds like you and Tom need to figure out how you're going to handle getting information about the weights. . . .

SUSAN: I'm not going to lie about it! And we didn't . . . we had said before . . . there wasn't a question about it before, why is there all of a sudden.

MOTHER: We didn't disc . . . we discussed that we were going to go by the clinic weight at the eating disorder clinic. We didn't discuss that we weren't going to know what it was. We never discuss. . . .

SUSAN: . . . Tom said that if you lie to us then . . . He didn't say, "We're going to have to hear from the doctors." No one ever said that and I don't. . . .

THERAPIST: All right, so . . . it sounds like there is some more work to be done on a plan of the point system. Umm, and when does Tom get back?

MOTHER: Tonight.

THERAPIST: Great. So, what's the plan for the next couple weeks? I know you two boys will continue to help your sister by finding ways to express your love and concern.

MOTHER: Well, hopefully our plan is, umm, that she's going to gain weight. That's what our hope is . . . is that she will bring her weight back up.

THERAPIST: Any things that you can think of that might be new? Any things that you and Tom have been thinking about that you might want to implement?

MOTHER: Well, we keep trying to encourage her that we would like to see her drink three cans of Boost a day with her food, but we're having a little trouble with that because she's . . . she refuses. . . .

SUSAN: I eat . . . I eat so much more food than that . . . I'd have only 4,000 calories a day if I did that.

MOTHER: But it had . . . it has so much more better nutrition than the other stuff. You're getting calories, but you're not getting good nutrition.

SUSAN: Do you want me to stop eating and drinking Boost?

MOTHER: No . . . but I want. . . .

SUSAN: Well. . . .

MOTHER: I don't think that that's such a terrible thing because you could do it for snacks or eat a Boost bar. You could do it for snacks and then one in the evening . . . it doesn't have to be around your meal time.

SUSAN: No, but I don't . . . if I have that in addition to a meal when I'm having like probably over 2,000 calories a day. . . .

THERAPIST: I want to encourage you not to argue about calories . . . because you know how that battle goes . . . the Alien comes in and does most of the talking. . . .

MOTHER: Anyway, we haven't gotten that far, so. . . .

THERAPIST: You have a goal, though, that's progress.

MOTHER: I just keep working on trying to get her nutrition . . . more nutritious, let's put it that way. Less on calories and more on nutrition.

The therapist continues in the preceding exchanges to support the parental efforts at refeeding and the sibling support of their sister. The therapist also still addresses the need for joint parental action, even though the father is not present in the session. The therapist continually returns the need for parental action to both parents by always remembering to include Tom in the discussion.

THERAPIST: And that's a great goal and . . . and you have some thoughts about it. It sounds like Susan doesn't agree with them. . . .

MOTHER: We're trying . . . we just keep trying.

THERAPIST: Now, let's go over the progress that you've made though . . . there is . . . I want to say that the last time the two of you were here, you guys sat next to each other and there was some tension around talking about weight and support. Remember that? There was like, uh, . . . you don't remember?

SUSAN: I remember.

THERAPIST: Did you guys . . . have you guys talked about that at all because you seem even. though you don't agree, you seem more comfortable with each other talking about it over the last couple . . . since I saw you 2 weeks ago.

MOTHER: We had, uh, we had a really nice visit on the way back from the eating disorder clinic last week. We kind of talked about a lot of different things and on different issues . . . I don't know.

THERAPIST: So it was just the two of you?

MOTHER: Yes. . . .

THERAPIST: So you had some time alone? Is that hard to get . . . sometimes?

MOTHER: Uh, sometimes, but we spend a lot of time together . . . we do a lot of things. It's just that sometimes when you're in the car . . . you just . . . you can't go away from it. You have to deal with it 'cause it's right there. It's not like you can get away from it. So sometimes I find that if you have something really serious you need to talk about that sometimes being in the car is a good place. I mean . . . obviously, not if it's going to be yelling and screaming and that kind of stuff, because that's not safe on the road, but sometimes it's good to be able to stay with it without distractions.

THERAPIST: And you stayed stable.

SUSAN: Yeah.

THERAPIST: That's a really positive thing.

SUSAN: I'm very stable.

THERAPIST: You stayed out of the hospital. It sounds like there's been no purging . . . that's positive. It sounds like you and Tom are working together and planning things . . . you've had some creative thoughts . . . that's working in general. Umm, let's see, what else positive? There's a whole list of things besides Boost pudding? (*some laughter*). Lunches out. You've been able to eat in restaurants together. . . .

SUSAN: We're going out tomorrow with a friend.

MOTHER: Yeah, we're going to a restaurant.

In the preceding interventions the therapist works to integrate the efforts both to refeed and to modify parental criticism of Susan. He identifies evidence of some progress and sets a conciliatory tone.

THERAPIST: That's wonderful. And it sounds also like, even though Tom's been away, you've been able to work together as parents and support each other still . . . while he's been away. Are you guys going to have dinner on the way home, uh . . . and meet Tom somewhere?

MOTHER: No, he'll be at home 'cause he was coming in at like 3:30. . . .

THERAPIST: I know he usually cooks, right?

SUSAN: He cooks a lot.

MOTHER: Not so much anymore 'cause I'm always home. It used to be that he used to cook because I would be at work and then I would come home, but now that I'm always home. . . .

SUSAN: I actually . . . I actually brought dinner because normally if we go through we stop at like fast food and they'd get something. . . .

MOTHER: We haven't been stopping at fast food, we've been stopping at Fresh Choice [a restaurant].

SUSAN: Well. . . .

MOTHER: Well, it's sort of fast food but sort of food that you could consider eating. But it's still . . . that's still difficult because there's a lot of food there and it's still uncomfortable. . . .

Closing All Sessions with a Recounting of Progress

THERAPIST: Well, I think you've . . . I'd say there's been a lot of progress. It is clear that you and Tom are working together, even though he has been away. Also that you and Susan are reaching out to one another more and that the Alien has been pushed out a bit more. It is also clear that your brothers continue to be supportive. Your family should feel good about this hard work.

The therapist closes the session with a summary and positive comment on the work done by individuals and by the family as a whole.

10

Beginning Phase II: Helping the Adolescent Eat on Her Own (Sessions 11–16)

Summary of Phase II

The patient's surrender to her parents' demands to increase food intake, accompanied by steady weight gain, as well as the parents' relief after having taken charge of the eating disorder, signal the start of Phase II of treatment. As was the case in Phase I, the therapist advises the parents to accept that the main task in Phase II of treatment is the return of their child to physical health. Addressing the eating-disorder symptoms remains central in the discussions, while continuing weight gain with minimum tension is encouraged. However, in this phase the therapist can begin to bring forward for review issues the family has had to postpone until now (e.g., puberty, peer relations, sexuality, etc.). The eating disorder has interrupted regular adolescent development; therefore, the therapist's task is to use treatment to facilitate a return to normal adolescent development. Although adolescent issues are addressed in Phase III of treatment, the therapist begins to make a transition to these matters toward the end of this phase. This review, however, occurs only in terms of the effect these issues have on the parents in their task of assuring steady weight gain.

In concert with the adolescent's own developing autonomy and with the family's success in managing Phase I of treatment, during

Phase II increased independence from the therapist and his or her interventions is warranted. Therefore, sessions during Phase II should be scheduled 2 to 3 weeks apart. The therapist continues to weigh the patient at the start of each session. In addition, the need for help in the process of handing control of food and weight issues is extremely variable, and the therapist may find that the number of sessions needed during this phase will vary between two and six.

The mood displayed by the therapist in Phase II is different from the somber and sad tone characteristic of most of Phase I. By the time the family moves into Phase II, the patient and her family should have demonstrated progress in terms of weight regain. This advance should be reflected in the therapist's mood when he or she embarks on this next step in treatment. In addition, unlike the more structured nature of treatment interventions concerning refeeding the adolescent up to this point, guidelines for the therapist's style and technique from here onward is less circumscribed. From a developmental perspective, the eating disorder can be seen as having "interfered" with the patient's normal adolescent development. Therefore, the therapist's task now is to help get the patient "back into" adolescence. It should be noted that the parents also need to get "back into" adolescence—that is, they need to examine their own lives with the view toward their daughter growing up. The specifics of this process are highly individualistic, and there is seldom a prescribed way to proceed. Instead, we will provide broad guidelines for therapeutic procedures that the therapist should begin to introduce toward the latter part of this treatment phase.

During this phase, and as the patient has managed to recover her weight loss, her attitude toward the therapist changes. Whereas the patient was more watchful, almost hostile, toward the therapist but also dependent on him or her during attempts at weight gain, her attitude may have changed now to one that is more friendly and accepting. If the parents have succeeded in refeeding their youngster, the therapist may have gained some prestige that should be used to facilitate negotiations of the new patterns of relationships in the family. That is, the parents should attend to working out their affairs, while the children are primarily left to their own devices to take care of their business. Toward the end of Phase II, as the patient has taken charge of her own eating once more, the therapist ought to demote him- or herself and allow the parents and children to assume a leading role in treatment that should enable them to amplify their rights, strengths, and skills in the remaining sessions. What must happen during this phase is the freeing of the patient from her eating disorder so that she is more able to deal with the challenges of adolescence, challenges she may have felt incapable of addressing before. Once aligned with her peers and free of self-starving behavior, the patient can begin to negotiate issues of puberty, peer relationships, psychological autonomy, sexuality, and so forth. It is also now that the parents may feel able to take a step back and watch their daughter address these issues herself.

How the Therapist Assesses the Family's Readiness for Phase II?

Given the preceding summary of Phase II of treatment, the following is offered as an approximation of the criteria that should be met in order to signal readiness for Phase II of treatment:

- Weight is at a minimum of 87% of ideal body weight.
- Patient is able to eat without undue cajoling by parents, that is, and parents report no significant struggles getting the patient to eat regular meals.
- Parents report that they feel empowered in the refeeding process, that is, the parents demonstrate a sense of relief that they can manage this illness.

How the Treatment Team Changes in Phase II

For Phase II the treatment team remains intact, that is, the family therapy team plus the consulting team. As the eating disorder dissipates, treatment begins to resemble regular family therapy for adolescence, and the involvement of the consulting team, for example, the pediatrician or the nutritionist, may become secondary. However, the reappearance of eating-disorder symptoms might still necessitate maintaining the active involvement of the consulting team. Therefore, all team members should be kept abreast of the patient's progress. The relationship among the family therapy team itself, though, remains essentially unchanged from Phase I to Phase II.

The major goals of Phase II of treatment are:

- To maintain parental management of eating-disorder symptoms until the patient shows evidence that she is able to eat well and gain weight independently.
- To return food and weight control to the adolescent.
- To explore the relationship between adolescent developmental issues and AN.

In order to achieve these goals, the therapist undertakes the following interventions:

1. Weighing the patient.
2. Continuing to support and assist the parents in management of eating-disorder symptoms until the adolescent is able to eat well on her own.
3. Assisting the parents and adolescent in negotiating the return of control of eating-disorder symptoms to the adolescent.
4. Encouraging the family to examine relationships between adolescent issues and the development of AN in their adolescent.
5. Continuing to modify parental and sibling criticism of the patient, especially in relation to the task of returning control of eating to the patient.
6. Continuing to assist siblings in supporting their ill sister.
7. Continuing to highlight the differences between the adolescent's own ideas and needs and those of AN.
8. Closing sessions with positive support.

Although the treatment goals are the same for all needed sessions of Phase II, the emphasis of each session changes as one moves toward the end of this phase. For example, sessions may start out very similar to those of Phase I, with weight gain being the primary goal, but the emphasis will shift toward weight maintenance as control over eating is handed back to the patient. Finally, the therapist will begin to focus more on adolescent issues as she or he makes a transfer from Phase II to Phase III.

Weighing the Patient

Why

As in previous sessions, continued close monitoring of weight using the weight chart is an important mechanism for providing feedback to the patient and family on their progress. As weight gain usually continues to be important, at least during the early part of Phase II, the process of weighing the patient is critical.

How

At this point, the patient and therapist should have developed some increased rapport such that the weighing process becomes increasingly acceptable. The intimacy of sharing the vulnerable information of weight change should lead to greater trust overall. As this phase begins, the adolescent is often interested in discussing her wishes to be rewarded for her compliance with parental demands for refeeding by gaining increasing control over eating once again. The therapist should be receptive to these wishes without committing him- or herself to a course of action in response to them, other than assuring the patient that the parental control of food and weight will eventually end. The weight chart documents progress toward this end and therefore provides an opportunity to help generate a realistic perspective on the achievements of the family to date. On the other hand, it is not enough to assume that all that is happening in treatment is related to the patient's weight gain, especially during this phase. So, as the phase continues, emphasis on the weight chart may decrease.

Continuing to Support and Assist the Parents in Management of Eating-Disorder Symptoms until the Adolescent Is Able to Eat Well on Her Own

Why

Weight gain remains fragile at the early stage of Phase II of treatment, and optimal weight has not yet been achieved. Therefore, the therapist has to make sure that the parents do not relax their vigilance insofar as the refeeding process is concerned. Although this task is very similar to that described in Phase I, the therapist should note the shift in emphasis here. Whereas until now the therapist's task was that of helping and coaching the parents to get their daughter to eat more, the therapist's role here shifts more toward that of greater delegation. That is, the therapist wants to consolidate the parents' trust in their own abilities to make appropriate decisions in the process of refeeding their daughter. This is particularly important as the next therapeutic task is to have the parents negotiate with their daughter how to return control over eating back to her. During this phase, questions about the patient's ability and level of exercise often arise. The best approach is one that focuses the question of caloric intake once again on what the patient's own body suggests—eat enough to have enough energy to exercise. Caution about possible injury during exercise because of osteopenia or osteoporosis also points to the need for continuing and consistent parental management of the patient's eating.

How

Similar to the therapist's regular review of the parents' efforts at refeeding their daughter that earmarked much of Phase I, the therapist should start this phase of treatment with the same goal in mind. The therapist will insist that the parents remain relentless in their efforts to restore normal weight until they are convinced that the patient no longer doubts their ability to prevent her from starving herself. The therapist has to show determination to "stay" with the eating-disorder symptoms in order to send a powerful message to the parents that, for now, refeeding is the focus of treatment. At every session, the therapist has to carefully review events surrounding eating and discuss weight gain (or lack thereof) with the family members. The family's strategies to bring about weight gain should dominate discussions for as long as it is appropriate. For instance, each family member should be asked about events of the past week and how they have gone about the task of refeeding. In the style of circular questioning outlined previously, each response should be verified with every family member in turn to determine how he or she would describe events. Discrepancies should be carefully examined, as their clarification helps the therapist to select and reinforce those steps the parents will have to take to improve their refeeding efforts. As before, the therapist should use these sessions to carefully bolster the parents in their knowledge of nutritious and high-calorie meals and to reinforce their efforts to bring about healthy eating and weight gain. It is also important at this point that the perspective of "what's in it for the patient" be remembered. This may mean taking particular note of what motivates the patient. In general, this means getting the patient back in school, in age-expected activities, and engaged with her peers.

Assisting the Parents and Adolescent in Negotiating the Return of Control of Eating-Disorder Symptoms to the Adolescent

Why

Once the patient is relatively free from the eating disorder, it is timely for the parents to allow the patient to assert her independence in this respect, which is part of the development of healthy adolescent independence. Also, the gradual phasing out of parental supervision should serve as a trial period to see whether the adolescent can cope with eating adequately on her own without the reappearance of eating-disorder symptomatology thwarting her progress.

The therapist's responsibility here is to assist the parents and the adolescent in bringing about a careful and mutually agreed-upon handing over of responsibility in this domain from the parents to the adolescent. This process is orchestrated against the backdrop of each family's unique rituals or habits of regular eating activities before the eating disorder changed the family's mealtimes. Although the parents may seek guidance from the therapist about how to proceed with handing control of eating back to the patient, it is ultimately the parents, in collaboration with the patient, who should decide how to proceed with this process. This is a delicate maneuver, as the therapist must balance the involvement of the patient, who might jump at the opportunity to regain responsibility in food choices, the parents, and her- or himself in terms of the decision-making process.

How

As stated previously, the task of refeeding (as described in Phase I) is continued during Phase II, although with a gradual change in emphasis. Soon in Phase II, the therapist will guide the family toward relinquishing their control over the patient's eating. This can only be done if the patient's weight has been mostly recovered and if the therapist is reassured that improvement will continue even when the parents begin to exert less vigilance. Parents may choose to gradually lessen their control over this process in several ways, for example, by letting the patient serve herself at mealtimes while the parents continue to supervise this activity. Alternatively, parents may allow the adolescent more of her own food choices, as long as these selections represent healthy and adequate quantities of food. Another way to move forward is for the parents to leave the patient to her own devices for one or two meals per day while still supervising the main meal. Ultimately, the parents and the patient would want to arrive at an age-appropriate decision that is in keeping with each family's unique set of rules about food shopping, food preparation, joint family meals versus individual responsibility and tastes, and so on.

Encouraging the Family to Examine Relationships between Adolescent Issues and the Development of AN in Their Adolescent

Why

Once eating ceases to be the focus of discussions, the therapist should engage the family in negotiating important adolescent issues that have been postponed until now. Overall, the patient should be pushed as much as possible and as soon as possible into age-appropriate socialization. This concern was postponed while the parents concentrated their efforts on the refeeding process. However, at this point the therapist should begin to assist the patient to negotiate adolescence and young adulthood without the eating disorder.

Until now, everyone in the family has had to focus primarily on the eating disorder. The role of the therapist now is to assist the family to begin the process of reengaging the outside world, that is, helping the adolescent to embark on the tasks of adolescence and the parents to negotiate their relationship in the absence of the eating disorder. Adolescents with an eating disorder are often childlike and asexual, are more socially isolated than their peers, and have limited opportunities for psychosexual development. At the same time, because of the eating disorder, parents may have become overprotective and too involved in the patient's life, further limiting healthy adolescent exploration. Depending on the age of onset, the eating disorder itself undoubtedly interfered with the patient's normal psychosocial and psychosexual development. For instance, adolescents with an illness such as AN are often undereducated about sexuality and restricted in their social contacts and may have various concerns about their bodies and their sexual attractiveness. The therapist can begin to address these issues in terms of the effect they have on the parents' task of ensuring steady weight gain. In addition, the therapist should begin to help the parents find time for themselves on a self-prescribed frequency.

How

An example of a situation in which these issues can begin to be explored within the context of a continuing focus on the eating disorder is adolescent dating. Although dating in itself is representative of many important issues in adolescent development, such as individuation and psychosexual maturation, the patient can successfully embark on this course only when eating is no longer of concern. At this point in treatment, the therapist does not discuss the bigger issue but rather concentrates on whether all concerned are reassured that the patient can go out for dinner with a friend and make appropriate food choices. The therapist should let the parents and patient problem solve in a session to work out a plan concerning choice of restaurant and the food items that will be ordered. This way, parental anxiety is diminished, and the patient does not feel the need to impress her date and can remain focused on nurturing her fragile recovery from her eating disorder.

Continuing to Modify Parental and Sibling Criticism of the Patient, Especially in Relation to the Task of Returning Control of Eating to the Patient

Why

The reasons that family criticism is suspected to contribute to poorer outcome were enumerated previously. In the context of Phase II, the issue of family criticism is more directly focused on the return of eating to the adolescent. There is a renewed opportunity for parents and siblings to reproach the adolescent with AN and thereby compromise her best efforts. This may undermine the patient's attempts to return to healthy eating and can trigger greater resistance to help from her family.

How

The basic mechanisms for modifying parental and sibling criticism were described previously. During this phase, especially as the adolescent is encouraged to take up eating on her own, the therapist can model approval and acceptance of her struggle by saying such things as, "Although you did not fully succeed in your efforts to eat on your own, it is clear that you made a good effort" or, alternatively, "It seems your parents have high expectations of you, and although part of you wishes to meet them, in other ways you may feel that you can never achieve them. This may frustrate you and them at times and lead to conflicts, although your goals are the same—that is, to help you get your life as a teenager back."

Continuing to Assist Siblings in Supporting Their Ill Sister

Why

Again, the basic reasons for this type of intervention were previously discussed. However, it may seem that at this point sibling support is less vital. The case has been made that siblings should support their ill sister, but because she is clearly getting better, they may feel their work is done. It is true that the need for their specific support in relation to helping the patient tolerate the refeeding efforts of her parents does diminish in this phase. Nonetheless, the adolescent has not yet recovered and still needs support, especially when she advocates for more autonomy. Siblings are still important in helping her to sustain herself during this process.

How

The strategies for involving peers were illustrated earlier. At this point, it is usually only necessary to continue to bring the issue up during every session. The therapist may inquire of each of the siblings, "What did you do that helped your sister feel better this week about herself?" It is helpful to explore in some detail both the thought behind the action and the ill adolescent's appreciation or lack of appreciation for the effort.

Continuing to Highlight the Differences between the Adolescent's Own Ideas and Needs and Those of Anorexia Nervosa

Why

It is important that the difference between the thoughts and goals of AN and those of the adolescent continue to be explored. During this phase, it is usually much clearer what these differences are. The rationale for this type of intervention was provided previously, but in this phase, the therapist should continue to be assured that the differences between AN thinking and the adolescent's own goals and aspirations are continuing to diverge.

How

The basic strategies were presented previously. However, in this phase, the therapist can emphasize the differences between the thinking and goals of AN and those of the adolescent through the negotiating process of regaining control of eating from the parents. Thus, the therapist encourages the adolescent to set her own goals for recovery—for example, returning to a dance class that AN deprived her of because of her severe malnutrition. In addition, the therapist should explore failure to achieve such goals as a way to invigorate the adolescent's own wish to differentiate herself from AN.

Closing Sessions with Positive Support

Why

As in previous sessions, the attitude of the therapist at the conclusion of the session is warm and generally congratulatory so that guilt, powerlessness, and feelings of inadequacy are minimized.

How

As in previous sessions, the therapist summarizes the main achievements of the family while footnoting the shortcomings. This is done ef-
ficiently but with warmth as the family leaves. The therapist may take
care to say good-bye to each family member as he or she leaves the
room in order that they continue to feel recognized and valued.

End-of-Session Review

As was the case for all sessions in Phase I of treatment, the lead therapist should continue to review each treatment session with the rest of
the team during Phase II. At the end of each session, the following
questions should be discussed with the rest of the treatment team.

Common Questions for Phase II

*What if the patient decides to show renewed resistance
to parents' efforts?*

Some patients, either due to prior experience of their menstrual cycles
or perhaps because of their intuition about the specific weight level
that brings on their periods, may resist any further weight gain as they
approach a certain critical weight. Under these circumstances, patients
may decide to show renewed resistance to the parents' efforts at
refeeding. The therapist should use this opportunity to create another
"crisis," that is, informing the parents of the medical complications of
persistent amenorrhea. The purpose of this maneuver is to raise their
anxiety and reinvigorate them in their refeeding attempts.

*What if the patient's weight progresses well but then reaches a
suboptimal plateau?*

Very similar to the preceding question, some patients may progress
well—even beyond a weight that brings on a return of menses—but
then halt any further weight gain and reach a plateau at a suboptimal
level. Again, this is an opportunity for the therapist to point out to the
parents that even though it may appear as if the original crisis has been
successfully negotiated, a suboptimal weight, if maintained, can have
unhealthy consequences both in terms of normal physical development and psychological maturation. It may be difficult for some therapists to imagine how to address the issue of menstruation specifically

within the family-as-a-whole context. Although this is a highly personal area, especially for an adolescent girl, it is important that the therapist find a way to bring up the issue that respects the privacy of the adolescent and that is not humiliating to her but that also allows identification of this area of health as an important goal for recovery.

What if the patient's weight begins to slide downward once parents become exhausted or less vigilant in their supervision of the adolescent's eating?

This would be a poor prognostic sign, and the therapist should reinvigorate Phase I strategies to guide the parents quickly toward reimplementing steps they took earlier to bring on weight gain. Often parents need to be reenergized to take appropriate action as, understandably, they have come to think the crisis has abated or they are exhausted with the task of refeeding. However, just as in Phase I, when the patient's weight gain may have been halted for reasons previously discussed, the therapist should alert the parents to the fact that weight loss can lead to chronic problems, such as infertility, osteoporosis, and so on. Weight loss at this stage of treatment is unfortunate and retards the progress of treatment while the therapist revisits previously tried weight-gain interventions.

What if the patient regains independence in eating and then starts losing weight once more?

This would be another poor prognostic sign. It is imperative that independence in eating is not prematurely returned to the patient. Although the choice of how to get the parents to relinquish control to the patient should ideally be worked out between the parents and patient, the therapist should dictate the timing, as well as the tempo, of this process. However, should the patient return to dieting after control over eating has been returned to her, it would demonstrate to everyone that this step was premature. The therapist should remotivate the parents swiftly and have them reestablish control over eating. The therapist and the parents should be careful not to appear punitive. After all, it is the therapist and parents who misjudged the patient's readiness to proceed without constant supervision of her eating. The therapist should note, however, that it is relatively uncommon for a return to starvation to occur if the transition to independent eating has been negotiated mutually and carefully. Once this temporary setback has been overcome and the handing over of feeding responsibilities to the patient has been successfully negotiated, the therapist returns to a focus on more general adolescent issues. However, in making the transfer from Phase II to Phase III, the therapist first concentrates on adolescent issues as they pertain to the refeeding process. For example, in this phase it would be appropriate to address how to manage eating outside the family home when with friends or on a date. The obvious issues here may be adolescent individuation and sexuality; these issues are the domain of Phase III. Still, the therapist ought to take note of the adolescent and family issues that may be touched upon here but that are addressed more thoroughly in the final phase of treatment.

What if the parents continue to rely on the therapist to solve problems?

Throughout treatment the therapist wants to reinforce the parents' ability to arrive at their own solutions to restore their daughter's weight. For most parents, this strategy reinforces parental refeeding abilities and independence in this regard. However, some parents may have come to rely on the therapist to solve these problems and may find it difficult to see themselves coping with their daughter's difficulties. In these cases, the therapist will use the few sessions in Phase II to help the parents problem solve in the sessions so that they may have the opportunity to arrive at their own solutions.

What if the therapist introduces adolescent themes too soon?

The therapist may be anxious to move treatment toward a different emphasis and may introduce adolescent themes at a time when weight restoration is still too tentative. The patient may see a diversion of attention away from the eating disorder as a potential opportunity to resume dieting attempts. This would be unfortunate, as it would signal the therapist to return once more to interventions appropriate to the first goal of this phase, that is, consistent parental management of eating-disorder symptoms, inevitably retarding the treatment process.

How does the therapist maintain his or her focus, keep the whole family engaged, and make a graceful move toward Phase III?

This can be a difficult part of treatment, as all parties concerned, both the family and the therapist, may be exhausted after months of maintaining a diligent focus on the eating-disorder symptoms. With the patient's weight all but returned to normal, the therapist may have to ward off his or her own desire, as well as that of the family, to curtail any further treatment. However, as we stated earlier, we believe that the eating disorder has disrupted normal adolescent development and that an essential part of successful treatment is to make sure that the patient is well on her way, with the help of her siblings and her parents, to negotiating adolescence once more. Although this may be a lengthy and involved process, the therapist has to make sure that the patient and the family do not return to previous ineffective and unhealthy ways to negotiate adolescent challenges. Instead, the therapist should use this opportunity to identify one or two key areas of adolescent development appropriate to the patient and her family and to put this forward for discussion in the final sessions of treatment.

Concluding Phase II

Most of the adolescent issues referred to until now are explored more thoroughly in the third and final stage of treatment. The patient's and the family's readiness to progress to Phase III is indicated when the patient's weight has been established and is being maintained between 90 and 100% of ideal body weight, when she eats regular meals without parental supervision, when the family is capable of discussing non-eating-related adolescent issues, and when the patient has been realigned with her peers.

11

Phase II in Action

*T*he following session illustrates a session relatively early in Phase II of treatment. In this example, the session unfolds in a manner predictable in a Phase II session, with increasing evidence that the problem of AN is being successfully countered, if not completely mastered.

Clinical Background

This is the family that was described in the vignette from Session 2. At this point, Rhonda's parents have been successful in taking charge of refeeding Rhonda but are not ready yet to turn eating back over to her. In this phase, the order of interventions is not proscribed. Instead, they are fluid and can be used more than once in a session as the need arises. In this family, there are no siblings, and parental criticism is especially low, so there are no examples of these interventions in this session.

To review, the major goals of Phase II of treatment are:

- To maintain parental management of eating-disorder symptoms until the patient shows evidence that she is able to eat well and gain weight independently.
- To return food and weight control to the adolescent.
- To explore the relationship between adolescent developmental issues and AN.

In order to achieve these goals, the therapist needs to undertake the following interventions:

1. Weighing the patient.
2. Continuing to support and assist the parents in management of eating-disorder symptoms until the adolescent is able to eat well on her own.
3. Assisting the parents and adolescent in negotiating the return of control of eating-disorder symptoms to the adolescent.
4. Encouraging the family to examine relationships between adolescent issues and the development of AN in their adolescent.
5. Continuing to modify parental and sibling criticism of the patient, especially in relation to the task of returning control of eating to the patient.
6. Continuing to assist siblings in supporting their ill sister.
7. Continuing to highlight the differences between the adolescent's own ideas and needs and those of AN.
8. Closing sessions with positive support.

Weighing the Patient

Rhonda is comfortable being weighed by her therapist and expresses pleasure in her progress. She notes that she believes she is doing better and feels that she is doing it more on her own. The session begins by going over the patient's weight chart. Weight gain has been minimal.

THERAPIST: Let's get started. How have the past 2 weeks been?

FATHER: Very good.

RHONDA: They said I was doing good at the clinic, so they cut my visits back to only once a week.

THERAPIST: What does "doing good" mean?

RHONDA: Gaining appropriate weight. I'm taking the medicine, not the medicine, but the calcium and stuff. I don't seem to be having problems, when they ask me questions, everything is fine, respiratory, heart, blood pressure, vitals, everything is good. That's what they're going by.

THERAPIST: That's good, because last time we talked, your weight had gone down. Have you gained it back?

RHONDA: What had gone down, yeah.

FATHER: Then she maintained, then she went up .4 kg, and that's when they cut her back. And she's been eating excellently.

In the preceding exchanges, the therapist reviews the weight progress to date. Because there has been less consistent progress, the therapist sets a more cautionary tone for the session in order to encourage the parents to keep engaged in the process of weight restoration.

Continue to Support and Assist the Parents in Management of Eating-Disorder Symptoms until the Adolescent Is Able to Eat Well on Her Own

THERAPIST: (*to parents*) Could you give me the doctor's report and the parents' report?

FATHER: Well, we see it because we're with her, and she's been eating very, very good, very healthy, and not skimpy portions, either. I noticed a huge difference in the past 2 weeks. When we left your office 2 weeks ago tonight, we didn't know where to go to get something quick to eat, so we went to Burger King. And at first Rhonda goes, "I'm going to have the Junior Whopper, but I want the large french fries and drink." So, I said, "Oh, good." So when she got up to the counter, she said, "I've changed my mind, I'm going to have the big Whopper." I was happy. She ate everything, ate everything, she's been really doing good.

MOTHER: She's been very conscientious about taking her calcium and zinc.

THERAPIST: That was a problem before?

MOTHER: No, she's always been. . . .

THERAPIST: Your concern last session was that she was backsliding?

MOTHER: That's because she wasn't eating enough, I don't think.

THERAPIST: That's right, you were able to see that, we need voices of reality, right?

MOTHER: Well, not only that but I noticed that she's been eating a little more each day, on her own, rather than us prodding her to eat. Occasionally, you know, we'll say, like a banana, she doesn't want to eat the whole banana; I'll say, "Well, you've had this much of it this time, so why don't you just go ahead and finish the rest of it."

In the preceding series of questions and comments, the therapist "checks in" with the parents about their level of anxiety concerning Rhonda's eating and weight problems and how they have responded to it. The therapist also endeavors to provide encouragement for their interventions that were successful. This helps the parents to stay with the task when it becomes more difficult.

RHONDA: And I still don't finish it, because I'd rather have more cereal than a banana, like I have a banana with my grandparents later, a whole one. Basically I want to eat half of one, but I'd rather have more cereal sometimes.

THERAPIST: So, from your point of view, you've given me an overview. How about from an inside of you (*to Rhonda*) point of view? Because last time you were struggling a little, remember? What happened, what's been going on?

RHONDA: Well, what's going on is that I'm eating good, I'm eating really good, I just keep counting the calories, but I'm eating good. So it's not that I'm counting the calories and eating poorly and making sure the calories are staying underneath a certain amount, but I'm keeping count of the calories. But I'm eating good.

THERAPIST: So, does it mean you would like not to keep track of the calories?

RHONDA: Well, I guess in a way I feel kind of not sure of myself if I don't keep count of that. I feel like I'm not, maybe, eating enough or eating too much.

THERAPIST: So, it's both.

RHONDA: But I wasn't really counting calories much before, but I am now. But as I see it it's in a good way because I'm eating.

THERAPIST: So you're making sure? How many calories do you think you need?

RHONDA: Maybe 2,500, 2,400 calories a day.

In the preceding exchange with Rhonda, the therapist turns to the patient for her input on her progress on food and weight issues. The therapist intends to support Rhonda's developing awareness of her control over her recovery and to gauge her ability to begin to take on more self-monitoring with less parental supervision. The tone is supportive without overidentifying with her problems. The therapist is keeping in mind that Rhonda's problems with weight and food are separate from Rhonda herself.

THERAPIST: (*to parents*) Do you agree? Because you had a good assessment last time.

MOTHER: I think it's getting close to that, I'm trying to kind of stay to some degree at bay, and watching her, keeping myself at bay.

THERAPIST: (*to Rhonda*) I don't understand what happened there?

RHONDA: Oh no, just the word, I haven't heard it before.

MOTHER: Keeping at bay, meaning, you know, to stay on the outside.

The therapist again turns to the parents for their impressions and to reinforce their overall responsibility for the weight gain and monitoring process at this point. The therapist moves back and forth between the parents and the child in this way to keep the family as a whole engaged, as well as to reinforce the important subsystems in the family structure.

Assisting Parents and Adolescents in Negotiating the Return of Control of Eating-Disorder Symptoms to the Adolescents

THERAPIST: Do you think she's ready for that? Let me say, the second phase of treatment, which you're entering, is sort of saying, she's eating enough, she's at a good enough weight. You feel like you can hand some responsibility back.

FATHER: Well, honestly. . . .

THERAPIST: If you do it carefully?

FATHER: We didn't have to do very much prodding in the last 2 weeks, actually very little.

RHONDA: I was pretty much eating on my own. I'm getting my calories, and I just feel safer if it's healthier food, you know, cereal, banana, bagel and jam, pasta, vegetables, fruit, maybe sometimes peanut butter and jelly, I have muffins too, I have Power Bars. I feel safer if I eat healthy foods.

THERAPIST: Are you eating healthy foods?

RHONDA: Oh yeah, occasionally we go to fast food, but I feel safer if it's healthier food, you know, pasta's healthy, fish maybe, chicken, maybe some meat, but I like Power Bars, I like Boost, I like bananas, I like vegetables.

MOTHER: That stuff is during the day.

RHONDA: Yeah, like pasta is the main dinner, or like fish or meat or something.

Although the therapist is interested in the opinions of both the parents and Rhonda, it is ultimately going to be the parents who need to make the decision about when Rhonda is ready to be more on her own. Both of the previous and some of the following interactions illustrate this balancing of interest with the ultimate parental authority that is key in this intervention.

THERAPIST: The question is about your readiness as parents to let Rhonda eat more on her own. Is she really ready to move on? Because here's what happens, you could give it a try and see how it's going. If it is too soon, things could go not so well. Now I think that is sort of what happened last time, maybe 3 weeks ago, when you were less vigilant. But at the same time, you do want her to get a chance to do it on her own, because that's the goal.

MOTHER: Well, I think she probably wants to do it on her own so we wouldn't bug her, we wouldn't prod her, we wouldn't keep on top of her that much, and she probably is very aware of what's she's eating. You know, she still probably is thinking calories, and going back to normalcy, if she didn't think calories, then psychologically she'd be better off if she could think of other things.

THERAPIST: Sounds like you're not quite sure if she's quite ready.

MOTHER: Not totally, but like I said I'm trying to. . . .

FATHER: Stay at bay.

THERAPIST: Stay at bay, that's right. But still watchful. Not too far away. You could get there and it would be hard to leave.

MOTHER: Exactly

THERAPIST: (*to father*) How about you, how are you feeling about all this? Sounds like you are a bit hesitant?

FATHER: Oh, yeah, honestly, I think she did great.

THERAPIST: She did do great.

FATHER: As long as she keeps it up and gets a promising report Tuesday from the doctors and the checker. "You know, gee, Rhonda, you gained a little more weight."

THERAPIST: That's what you want to see, right, because she's not at the exercise weight level, because she wants to ride her horse.

RHONDA: Oh, they probably wouldn't want me to. They say 15 minutes of exercise. I don't exercise.

THERAPIST: That's where you start, you are going to add to that if you stay stable.

RHONDA: But I don't like, but I don't like exercising, I think it's boring. The only thing I do is horseback riding, which they consider exercise, I'm sure. But ring work is when you're in a ring and you're exercising, like you're posting, which is going up and down, you're . . ., you're doing all that. But, I don't have access to that at this point. I just have access to trails and whatever, so needless to say I can only walk. Which I use my leg muscles to stay on, but you can't do much more than that.

THERAPIST: Falling off is a hazard, too.

MOTHER: Especially with her bones.

RHONDA: But I mean that also.

THERAPIST: Did they check your bones?

RHONDA: They haven't rechecked them.

THERAPIST: But when they checked them?

RHONDA: There was a deficiency, that's why they have me on 24 mg of calcium a day, and they want me to retake it next January.

THERAPIST: It takes awhile to replenish your bones. You don't want to fall off. Even if you ride well, it doesn't matter, your bones are very fragile at this point.

In the preceding series of exchanges, the therapist attempts to illustrate the need for continued weight gain for physical health both to the parents and to Rhonda. Illustrating this through specifics about possible osteoporosis, as well as other health hazards, is a key element in keeping the family focused on eating and weight gain, even when Rhonda is doing somewhat better. This keeps the pressure on and hopefully leads the family to be cautious about letting up on their monitoring prematurely. These observations also are made to help Rhonda understand some of the reasons that she may still need to submit to her parents' authority for the time being in the area of weight and food monitoring.

RHONDA: Well, Christopher Reeve, he rode well. Well, he was jumping. I don't, I tried it for awhile, jumping, but I wasn't real secure with that. So at this point I can't even, I can't do anything to work. But the horse gets enough work, I guess, with hills or whatnot.

THERAPIST: I would like to help your parents to figure out when they feel you might be able to try eating more on your own. How much do you need to gain until you can exercise?

RHONDA: One pound, I guess, because I'm at 42.7 kilos, I need to be at 44.

THERAPIST: What was your discharge weight?

RHONDA: 43.

THERAPIST: So the kinds of things you are going to be looking for as parents are her readiness, so you can stop encouraging her.

MOTHER: Prodding her.

THERAPIST: Prodding her is something you do to ensure that there will be a consistent pattern to getting her to eat what she needs.

RHONDA: Well, they haven't prodded me at all because I eat.

THERAPIST: So they're not bothering you when you don't eat?

RHONDA: Well, they haven't had to at all because I eat what I need.

FATHER: Not in the past 2 weeks we haven't.

MOTHER: What I usually do is, like, when we're preparing dinner, I just happen to ask, "Well, what did you have for lunch today, or your snack?"

THERAPIST: And Rhonda tells you what she'd like to eat?

RHONDA: Well, my dad, I ask him if he wants to dish it out.

THERAPIST: You're still dishing it out.

FATHER: Umm, not really, because if Rhonda says "I want to do my own" we let her, and we watch her. Like last night she ate her meal, she had a big dish of fresh vegetables and Italian pasta, and she finished it, and I said, "Well, I really don't know if I want any more," and my wife said the same thing. I said "Well, what about you, Rhonda?" She says, "I do want some more." So I was a little surprised at that and what I did, I said, "Do you want me to dish it out or do you want to take what you want?" she said, "No, you dish it out for me," so I did, and what we did was, we showed it to her first. I said, "Does this look okay, can you finish this?" and she said, "Yeah, I can," and she finished every bit of it.

THERAPIST: So that was sort of a compromise. You looked at the amount and it looked okay. You (*the parents*) were in control, but she could say, "Too much" ?

In the preceding exchanges, the therapist explores with the family in what ways they are currently monitoring Rhonda's intake. The therapist looks for evidence about how closely the parents are monitoring her and identifies in the last exchange that the parents are now more comfortable negotiating with Rhonda than before about what she needs to eat.

FATHER: She surprised us when we went to breakfast one morning, over the weekend. We went to a French café. And she says, "I'm going to have a bowl of cereal and bring a Boost with me." They came to the table and it was a huge bowl of cereal, and she put Boost in it, and then she ordered a vegetarian omelet, which had roasted red potatoes, and a muffin with it. And I say she only left about a third of the omelet. She ate all the cereal and the Boost, two-thirds of the omelet, the potatoes, and her muffin, and a cup of coffee, and I was shocked.

MOTHER: Oh, and she had a glass of juice.

FATHER: A glass of juice, and I was shocked.

THERAPIST: Shocked or happy?

FATHER: Very happy, because we didn't have to tell her to eat, we were just watching her eat. "Oh, this is delicious."

THERAPIST: (*to Rhonda*) Was it good?

RHONDA: Yeah, that was like 2 weeks ago.

MOTHER: But, what we do is, we don't jump for joy when she eats a lot, or we don't get real angry when she doesn't eat a lot, we just act like normal.

THERAPIST: That sounds like it has been helpful. It looks as if you have recovered the weight you lost a few weeks ago. And your plan is to get the rest of them?

RHONDA: Oh, the rest of my kilos, yeah. That's only .3 kilos or so. . . .

FATHER: I'll say she'll get at least that.

MOTHER: She probably will surpass her discharge weight.

THERAPIST: That's terrific for everyone.

The therapist in the preceding exchanges provides positive reinforcement for the work that the family and Rhonda have done to regain the weight she lost since the last session. Although the therapist is aware that there is more work to be done, the strategy of consistent and persistent reinforcement for accomplishments helps the family to persevere.

RHONDA: I hope they [her pediatric group] will let me begin exercising soon. I'm surprised they don't consider going up to the horse and brushing or taking care of his exercise, because it is basically. Because it's a big animal.

THERAPIST: Maybe they don't know, huh?

RHONDA: No, they do because I talk to them and I tell them I go and I groom and I spend time with him, and they know it's a big animal, I mean he's huge, he's 16 hands, that's not huge but. . . .

FATHER: He's big, he's big to me. You know about horses, too, then?

THERAPIST: You know the group doesn't want to prevent you from having time with your horse, they really want you to be able to be with, even if they recognize that there may be some exercise involved, they don't want to deprive you. That's not the model they have. I guess if they thought you were running around him in circles, or doing ring exercises with him, then I think they wouldn't want you to do that. They really ultimately want you to be happy. I know it doesn't always feel that way, but we all do really want you to be happier.

RHONDA: Well, that makes me happy. You know I'm up there, not every day, probably every other day on average.

Continuing to Highlight the Differences between the Adolescent's Own Ideas and Needs and Those of Anorexia Nervosa

THERAPIST: Well, I know that's one of your goals, and I want to integrate that into thinking about what comes next. It's a real turnaround. Why, do you think? Because we were all worried only 2 weeks ago. It looked really promising after the hospital, then there was a period of less optimism. (*To parents*) What have you done?

RHONDA: Well, they haven't done anything, I have. They haven't done anything. It's probably been because lately I have been so happy, so happy with my horse. You know, he has just pleased me so much that it's unbelievable, because when I started really going up there . . . the first time I went up there when I was leaving, I was waving and he started making noises that horses make, like "Oh, come back." And that made me feel good. So I kept going back, and then when he started seeing me, he started making noises when I'm just back there way back at the barn, and I'm talking like an idiot to myself, "Wait, did I forget something?" You know, it's like he hears me, then when I come around, I peek around the corner, he's standing there, and he starts to make some noise, and his ears are up. You know, it just makes me happy. And I'm just concentrating on him.

THERAPIST: It's something other than food and weight to focus on.

RHONDA: Well, yeah, I'm still focused on calories, but that's something separate from school, I don't let it get in the way of school. You know some people look at calories to a certain extent, some people it may be just trying to eat healthy, they think they eat too much fast food or, I don't know. But I'm doing real good in school actually. I took my last final to make up, and I think I did really good on that.

THERAPIST: You've caught up on your schoolwork then?

RHONDA: Yeah, it was just one page of questions.

FATHER: She's been focused, very focused.

THERAPIST: (*to Rhonda*) It's easier when you're not worried about food and weight all the time, isn't it?.

MOTHER: Last night when she came home from the horse, she had a couple of good things to talk about. Her father spent a long time with her and explained everything. She's now really getting focused in to taking care of the horse now, and she likes the relationship. And she explained that a representative from the junior college visited, and she has already filled out an application, not so much for the school, but to take a tour in April, and to talk to a counselor. So her goal is to take the courses she needs so she could be eventually transferred to a 4-year college, because she wants to do that. So she's really focused on that, too.

In the preceding exchanges, the therapist works mostly with Rhonda to separate her from the illness in terms of identifying things she wishes to accomplish besides weight loss and being thin. In her case (and in most), the patient has a number of important other aspirations and concerns. One of the ways the therapist can stay aligned with the patient, even when he is encouraging the parents to go against the patient's overt wishes not to gain weight or eat, is by tracking these other interests and concerns insofar as they are affected by the eating disorder. In this way, the therapist is able to keep a relationship with the patient, who might otherwise feel unattended to.

THERAPIST: Right, so, what do you (*to parents*) think?

FATHER: Well, actually, it is like Rhonda says, we really didn't do anything, we monitor. Because we're watching, and we're doing what, we're prepared to do what you told us to do, but it really seemed in the last 2 weeks we did not have to step in, and I feel as if Rhonda was doing this on her own, and we're watching everything she's eating, and she's eating a good amount of food. I don't want to step in and antagonize her, because I'm afraid she could get withdrawn again, and say, well, I don't know how this illness really works, and I like what I saw.

THERAPIST: That's great! (*To parents*) You are assessing the situation, if things weren't going well, you'd see that, you weren't even risking that, I'm assuming. (*To Rhonda*) You get to be a little more independent. You're getting your independence back around an area that you've had to be more dependent on your parents.

FATHER: And what we always do is, when she eats a meal, and she eats good portions, we tell her, "You ate very well tonight, or today." We always tell her that we're pleased. We always praise her on that, too.

RHONDA: Well, that's fine, but they never praised me before.

FATHER: Oh, yeah, we did.

RHONDA: But not when I would, but not when I would, you know, not like . . . or something, but that's okay.

Again, in the preceding exchanges, the therapist is working with the parental subsystem to emphasize that their assessment of the situation is of ultimate importance and to praise them for their attempts.

THERAPIST: Does it bother you that they are pleased? They have some respect for the illness, they've seen it at its worst, and you've come back.

RHONDA: No, it doesn't bother me. Yeah, I think that something that may seem really small, but something that could have been getting me down too, was I felt really frustrated in the beginning with my horse, and that could have been getting me down, too. Because at times I felt, at times, like, I'm never going to get used to him. He's big, he's not listening, he's not doing this right, he's not doing that, but then once things just seemed to start falling into place, and I felt like he was recognizing me to be his companion, and not Mary—which is the owner of the place where we are boarding him—and not her as his companion, which is probably what he thought for awhile, it makes me feel better, it makes me feel more responsible for him, and makes me feel like, you know, just recently I feel like, he's mine. It's not just like I'm going riding somewhere, and then I leave, and then he's used for other lessons. I'm in control of who rides him, and I have the say.

THERAPIST: Did you get him right when you went into the hospital?

RHONDA: Two weeks before.

THERAPIST: So, you really hadn't had time to work with him.

RHONDA: No, I only had him 2 weeks, and I didn't have really time to ride him, the weather was lousy. I went up there, I groomed him real quick, then I had to go because it was getting dark early. Sometimes I felt like, I don't know how to deal with this because I've never had my own horse before, it seemed at times an overwhelming responsibility.

FATHER: But, you've worked around horses.

RHONDA: Yeah, but I've never owned a horse, so it was a different kind of. . . .

THERAPIST: It's different to feel responsible for him.

RHONDA: Yeah, it's just something that I'm really proud of. When I go up there it's like 2 hours fly by. I bring, there is this little stool that he likes to knock over, and he thinks it's funny. I bring it up there, and I bring a book, and I sit there and I read. Sometimes he comes over and slobbers on my hand and stuff.

FATHER: We actually bought the horse for Rhonda as an incentive, because she had not been hospitalized yet. But, it was back and forth to the doctor, the medical doctor, and we knew that she had a problem, and we were, this is before she even knew about the children's hospital or anything. . . . We always knew that she would love to own her own horse, and we discussed it and said, "If we bought her the horse, gave her something to look forward to and everything, maybe this would bring her out of it." And it only did for about 2 weeks, and we noticed she went complete opposite, and we thought, "We're in trouble now." At that point is when Nancy . . . caught her in the middle of tests and everything and said, she has to be admitted to the hospital.

MOTHER: In fact, her father and I were just talking last night, about how Rhonda was so frustrated that she didn't like being around the horse, she can't control him, she doesn't like this or that. And then, we were upset at that time hearing this. And I told her father last night, the whole reason behind it was that, Rhonda, she was only like 84 pounds, she didn't have any energy, she didn't have any stamina, and she had no nutritional value getting into her body, so naturally she couldn't control the horse or take care of it, so that's why it affected her psyche as well as her body, so that's why she felt the way she did. Now that she's stronger, and she's better psychologically, she deals with stuff differently.

In the preceding exchange, the therapist works with the entire family, but especially with Rhonda, to explore a strategy they employed to try to encourage Rhonda to eat. In this case, the strategy did not work. The therapist does not dwell on this failed attempt, but instead moves ahead to other attempts.

THERAPIST: One of the things we talked about last time, was the two of you, you have different skill bases that you can use together to help Rhonda. For example (*to mother*), you had a very clear understanding of how many calories Rhonda was eating. And you were very articulate about it as well. I asked you to explore that, in these 2 weeks a little bit, so you would have information from each other to work together. Did that come up at all? Was it important at all?

FATHER: I still don't know that much about calories.

THERAPIST: So, you didn't, you didn't check in with her and say, "Is she doing okay?" you just, you thought she was.

FATHER: Well, by seeing what she was consuming. . . .

THERAPIST: You thought she was.

FATHER: I didn't think, I knew, because I knew what she was eating. Because I know some of the things that she sat down, like even after eating a meal, she'll sit down and take out ice cream or chocolate cookies, and I said, "Well, I know." And especially the cookies we had at home, I know are very high in calories.

THERAPIST: One of the examples you gave was bringing ice cream and Rhonda refusing to eat any.

FATHER: Yes, I remember that.

THERAPIST: What I'm trying do is to keep the two of you aware that in monitoring her, you both have something to offer her. You can still work together in terms of making sure that you're both on the same page in terms of how she's doing.

FATHER: Well, we always are.

THERAPIST: That's great, how do you know that?

MOTHER: I kind of changed my, not my attitude, but my action. I stand back, and I observe very closely, it's like a silent observation. And I haven't been forcing Rhonda to do anything. And Gary was telling me last night, let's not dwell on any type of situation to make her eat or anything, let's just, you know, do it normally. Because otherwise, she'll just start withdrawing, and she'll just rebel and not eat, so I've been pretty cognizant about it, and I've been trying not to say too much.

In the preceding exchanges, the therapist follows up on roles and specific competencies that the parents have identified for each other to help them in monitoring and supporting Rhonda's weight gain and food intake. The therapist attempts to clarify for the parents what they are doing and the decisions they are making, as well as to reinforce that they are working together to combat this illness.

RHONDA: And I know how you'd react, you say, "No, you need to step in." I know that's how you'd react, I've seen you react that way, but in a way. But it won't make me withdraw, I could see if I was maybe on the borderline or whatnot. I could see where that may make me withdraw then, but it won't make me withdraw if they step in because honestly I could say . . . You know, knock on wood, I'll stay like this.

Encouraging Family to Examine Relationships between Adolescent Issues and the Development of Anorexia Nervosa in Their Adolescent

THERAPIST: (*to Rhonda*) Sounds like you're thinking more about the future without anorexia?

RHONDA: Honestly, I could say that I'm too happy to withdraw, just with information I'm hearing about colleges, it just makes happy and more secure, that I'm hearing, that I'm going to a junior college and about the 4-year college. And they used an example of College X, that the person who is transferring from a 2-year, is preferred over someone else that might be transferring from a 4-year. That they are already in, they are just switching colleges, and, you know, it just makes me feel more secure. They don't care if you didn't really do good in high school, they are giving you a chance to start over, which is what I need, and do really good in junior college, and if you do well there, you can transfer to the 4-year college, so you have a chance to start over if you aren't doing really good in high school.

THERAPIST: So, you're feeling more optimistic about life, that there are other things and hopes and dreams?

RHONDA: Yeah, now that I know I surpassed, overcoming any fear, any overwhelmingness of the horse. Once I know I surpassed that, I then saw that I was safer with college and everything. Now I feel like I can go ahead and see what I'm going to do in the future.

FATHER: That's part of, you're saying, that this is starting to break away. It's coming apart now.

THERAPIST: That's what it seems to me, like, it seems like you're moving away from anorexia. You're no longer only focused on food and calories . . . there are still some concerns about calories. It's not going to be totally easy all the time, but it's a lot better than it was, because there is a lot more of you and what you want to be showing. There's the Rhonda who wants to do well in school, wants to have time with the horse, wants to plan for her future in a junior college, and then a 4-year. Those are things that are beginning to blossom and couldn't before. And you're right, if those things continue to hold sway, the eating disorder is going to be held at bay and maybe become obscured itself.

The therapist again moves back to Rhonda in these exchanges, attempting to balance his interest and attention to both subsystems. In the first phase of treatment, a great deal of emphasis is on the parents and getting them working well together and effectively on the problem of refeeding their daughter. In the third phase of treatment, the emphasis is more on the daughter and her adolescent process. In this second phase, the therapist must be committed to a middle course that moves back and forth between the subsystems with almost equal time devoted to both until it becomes clear where the emphasis needs to be. The therapist sets the stage for exploring how Rhonda's planning for a more independent life as a college student may have been sabotaged by AN and how the family can move beyond this.

MOTHER: Well, Rhonda is a very intelligent person, she has a lot of common sense, she knows that if she wants to attain her goals and look toward the future, she knows she has to be healthy and eat nutritionally, and eat well, and be psychologically well, too, and to attain that, she has to eat well. So if she wants those goals, she'll do what she can to meet them. And I know she's smart enough to realize that "I better start eating well," and continue to do this, and be in upswing mode to get better, so she can reach those goals.

RHONDA: As far as this, the goal I want is more muscle. See, thinness isn't muscle, see when you're gaining weight back, from being how I was, too thin, all skin and bones, what you're gaining back, you don't have any muscle, you're gaining back all fat. What I want is muscle. Once you gain back weight, I want to turn it into muscle, because when you ride, you're using legs, you're using your inner thigh, you're using your outer thigh, you're using everything. And I want muscle. When I rode a year and a half ago, I had solid legs. I was eating a good breakfast and an excellent dinner and everything, and I was probably 105 or something, but I had muscle. And that's what I want, is I want muscular legs. I was looking at the movie, I'm sure you know it, *Striptease*, with Demi Moore, and Burt Reynolds. Demi Moore, she has, you could tell she worked out, because she has, her thighs were not small, they're actually rather big, but you could tell they are muscle mass.

FATHER: You could tell she's healthy.

RHONDA: You could tell she works out. I mean I wouldn't get thighs like that because I don't like to work out, but I would get solid thighs instead of like Jell-O, they would be solid, and that's what you get from riding.

THERAPIST: So, that's what we're aiming for. Have you talked to your pediatrician about that? Usually you can do 15 minutes to start, and then you can increase it by 15 minutes. So that pretty soon, over a month, you have about an hour.

RHONDA: Well, like 2. Because it takes about half an hour to go to the park, you want to ride an hour there, and a half hour back.

MOTHER: And also it takes time to tack them up, that's using your arms and everything.

FATHER: That's using muscles, you're right, because the saddle is not light.

THERAPIST: Do you ride Western or English?

RHONDA: Well, I don't care which way, I like them both, I've ridden both, bareback, too. But the reason I chose English is because, I don't jump or anything, but because the saddle is lighter. The Western saddle is way too big for me to get up on to the horse. So I needed something that is reasonable for me to lift up because I'm short, yeah, because I'm short.

THERAPIST: Do you want to do more general exercise?

RHONDA: One thing is I've never been wanting to exercise, I don't know, maybe because, I don't know, I think it's boring. Some people, they really enjoy it, they like lifting weights and working out, but I just don't find it fun. I find it fun riding, but that's because that's what I enjoy, obviously.

THERAPIST: Well, there's exercise, and there's exercise. So, something to anticipate, you're not quite there yet, is how exercise is going to change your caloric needs. If you exercise for a couple hours, riding, you use more calories. True, it may change the ratio of the fat to muscle, but you may still need more. It won't mean that because you're heavier, you're bigger.

RHONDA: Muscle weighs, like, if I was the same, say I was 105, with like just fat, I would probably weigh, if I was the same size, but I was muscle instead of fat, but I was the exact same size, I would probably weigh 110. I don't know if I would weigh more, because muscle weighs more, it's heavier, it's more solid.

MOTHER: My main concern now is that she starts getting her period, that she gains enough weight so to produce her estrogen, so she can start getting her period.

THERAPIST: I agree with that concern. How many months has it been?

RHONDA: Since August.

THERAPIST: Usually, it takes a certain amount of body fat to start the menstrual cycle again.

RHONDA: Two weeks ago my body fat was 13% or so.

MOTHER: I remember after her first hospitalization, her body fat was at like 9%.

THERAPIST: So, that's a really good gain, but it may have to be 18 to 25%

RHONDA: When I had my period, probably. I mean I don't know because I never had an accurate scale, and I never really knew if the scale was right or wrong, but I'm guessing it was on about maybe 98, 99. It was probably a little lower than 100. But honestly I don't know.

THERAPIST: Not having a period also affects your health, your bones, for example. Are you looking forward to having your menses return?

RHONDA: Yes, yes and no. More yes than no. Well, because, no, because it's a pain in the neck, but yes, because it's natural, it's something you have to go through, and eventually I'll lose it again, when I go through menopause, but that's not for awhile, so. . . .

MOTHER: That's not for a long while.

RHONDA: Yeah, but I want it because, you know, you have to have it to have kids, so. . . .

THERAPIST: Yes, yes, not just to have kids, but for your whole body to work well and be healthy. Were your periods difficult for you in some way?

RHONDA: No, I don't get cramps or anything.

THERAPIST: I know it's sort of a personal area, it is a personal area. But on the other hand, it is a part of medical progress.

FATHER: That's what we were saying, that we'll really rejoice when she gets her period back, because that's how her body is saying that she's healthy enough to make her period. . . .

MOTHER: That she can reproduce.

FATHER: Right, and come back.

RHONDA: That's how it was explained to me, if you were not eating enough, or making yourself sick, then your body is saying, "Well, there is something wrong in the environment, you can't bring any more kids into the world." So, I guess, it just stops the cycle.

In the preceding series of exchanges and interventions, the therapist once again identifies and emphasizes the need for further weight gain due to medical problems secondary to Rhonda's current low weight. The special emphasis on regaining menses is important, but it may cause some practitioners to take pause. It is uncommon to discuss a teenage daughter's menstrual status with fathers and younger siblings (especially brothers) in the room in the United States (though this is not true in other countries) and may be culturally so foreign in some groups that it is ill advised to have this type of discussion with all family members present. At the same time, the need to discuss and identify this key indicator of recovery and of adolescence cannot be bypassed. Therapists will need to find a way to undertake such a discussion that is at once respectful of the patient's privacy, family structure, and culture. The even tone and matter-of-fact approach used here may be appropriate as a middle course for many American families.

Closing Sessions with Positive Support

THERAPIST: It's true. Well, let's think about and wrap up this session and talk about it. What I've heard is Rhonda is really on the illness, really fighting it. It started that very night after our last session. Although no one has acknowledged that it was important work in that last session, it was important work. It really was. Rhonda saw it.

FATHER: You mean the session?

THERAPIST: The last session.

FATHER: I think everything combined, with the hospital and the therapy, is playing the biggest role in this.

MOTHER: You're here for moral support and guidance.

THERAPIST: I think you guys are doing the work, though. My point is, yeah, we're here, helping every way we know how, for moral support, for some ideas, for direction, for nets if things aren't going well, all of that. But something has happened in the last 2 weeks, starting at the end of the last session. You ate a Whopper and giant fries, and I think it just kept going in that direction. You have given me some really wonderful ideas on your internal perspective as well. You have gotten connected with parts of your life that were having to be deferred. But also the two of you have really gotten on board about it, and monitored carefully, and Rhonda has accepted that monitoring pretty well for now and wants it. And sometime in the future, relatively near future, you'll be able to move on to other kinds of issues. You'll notice I don't let us get into too much, until, really, this weight and eating disorder are a little bit farther, it's still the focus. So I think I will see you in 2 weeks. At the same time.

The therapist concludes the session by summarizing as many positive things that the patient and her parents have accomplished in the past weeks and during the session as possible. The tone is optimistic and encouraging.

12

Starting Phase III: Adolescent Issues (Sessions 17–20)

*I*n this chapter, we discuss the goals, interventions, and timing of Phase III. In addition, we present a general discussion of adolescent development and AN to serve as a general introduction to the overall types of issues that are addressed in this phase. Finally, we focus on how termination of this type of therapy is managed.

The third phase is initiated when the patient achieves a stable weight, the self-starvation has abated, and control over eating has been returned to the adolescent. The central theme here is the establishment of a healthy adolescent–parent relationship in which the illness does not constitute the basis of interaction. This entails, among other things, working toward increased personal autonomy for the adolescent, establishing appropriate intergenerational family boundaries, and recognizing the need for the parents to reorganize their life as a couple after their children's prospective departure. Attention to parents' professional and leisure interests are a legitimate focus of this phase.

Because the adolescent–parent relationship no longer requires the symptoms as an idiom of communication, discussion of other adolescent issues, such as independence, leaving home, and sexuality, may now be conducted. Each family will present with its unique issues, and it is the family who will put forward the agenda for discussion.

Often the therapist has to help parents learn that they can take care of themselves, that they can seek their own paths as a couple and as individuals, and that they do not need children as the reason for their existence. The aim of these final sessions is not to resolve these matters but to help the parents communicate to their children that these matters are the parents' business and that they, as a couple, will attend to them.

Readiness for Phase III

In this brief phase, the therapist and parents become convinced that the eating and weight disturbances and other symptomatic behavior will no longer occur and therefore are no longer the focus of discussion. However, the fear that the eating disorder may resurface is encouraged, and although the patient may still be somewhat preoccupied with worries about food, weight, and shape, these areas can be explored in a more relaxed atmosphere. The patient's weight is under control (approximating 90–100% of ideal body weight), and the responsibility for eating has been handed back to the patient.

The technique employed in this brief series of sessions builds on the increasing autonomy of the patient and the family from the therapist that has evolved during the previous two phases of treatment. That is, the family sessions are spaced at greater intervals (4–6 weeks apart), and the family is expected to be more able to take on the general problems of adolescence than it would have been previously, when the symptomatic expressions of AN dominated the family. In this sense, the family (as well as the patient) is really ready to take on the issues of adolescence as a developmental process supporting the ultimate autonomy and emancipation of the adolescent from the control of the parents.

In contradistinction to the portentous, brooding, and grave manner that characterized the initial sessions, the mood is comparatively optimistic, hopeful, and anticipatory. Because of their successful efforts at refeeding, the family can now be hopeful about their daughter's success in adolescence. This is not to say that there will not be a sense of loss or even mourning about the change of status of their daughter from child to young adult; in fact, this may indeed be one of the themes that will need to be explored. The brighter mood of these sessions supports the family's competence to take on the continuing challenges of adolescence.

The therapist's relationship with the patient has always been supportive while carefully separating the patient from the symptomatic expression of AN. In this phase the therapist must ensure that the patient's growing need for the autonomy she deserves is amply supported. This is possible if the therapist has succeeded in the earlier sessions in not alienating the patient and in underscoring the need to focus on her, as well as on the parents, during those sessions. In order for this phase to work, it is important for the therapist to build on and enhance this earlier alliance.

Because this phase is brief, only a few major themes can be worked on directly in the therapy sessions. This feature encourages the family and therapist to prioritize the most important issues to work on during sessions while acknowledging other issues that may be considered by the family outside of the sessions themselves. In this sense, this phase is targeted family therapy for adolescents who have recovered from an episode of AN. Weighing patients is not considered a core feature of this phase because it is assumed that these concerns are no longer central to the therapy.

The major goals for Phase III of treatment are:

- To establish that the adolescent–parent relationship no longer requires the symptoms as an idiom of communication.
- To review adolescent issues with the family and to model problem solving of these types of issues.
- To terminate treatment.

In order to accomplish these goals, the therapist undertakes the following interventions:

1. Reviewing adolescent issues with the family and modeling problem solving of these types of issues.
2. Involving the family in "review" of issues.
3. Checking how much the parents are doing as a couple.
4. Delineating and exploring adolescent themes.
5. Planning for future issues.
6. Terminating treatment.

Primer on Adolescent Development and AN

Background on general adolescent development and on the impact of illness on this process can assist the therapist in undertaking this phase. Adolescence can be conceived of as consisting of three stages, each of which has a specific relationship to development and behaviors. The first of these is the early stage (ages 12–14), which is primarily concerned with the dramatic physical changes associated with puberty. Getting this physical aspect of adolescence back on track has been the main focus of the first two phases of this manualized treatment. The middle stage of adolescence (ages 14–16) is dominated by the increasing influence of peers and developing abstract thinking abilities adolescents use to distinguish themselves from parents. The late stage of adolescence (ages 16–19) is associated with setting patterns and plans for work and establishing patterns of more intimate interpersonal relationships. These last two stages are more likely to be the central themes of the therapy during Phase III, though issues of body weight and shape may still arise.

In the early phase, the most significant issues concern changes associated with puberty itself. These are specifically related to issues of attractiveness, size, and maturational rate and their relationship to self-esteem and body image. These issues are sometimes processed somewhat differently by girls than by boys, at least in our culture. Girls generally are more concerned with maturing too early, being overweight or too tall, and not being perceived as attractive. Boys, on the other hand, are more concerned with maturing late, being too small or too short, and not being strong enough. For those who are recovering from AN, there may be evidence of difficulty accepting the adolescent body, and, even when they are weight recovered and eating well on their own, issues about how acceptable their bodies are likely to remain.

In the middle stage of adolescence, concerns related to peer relationships intensify. General themes of this period include dating competence, sexual orientation, and exploratory sexual experiences. Other issues, which may complicate development in this period, revolve around separating from family and include guilt, fears of abandonment, and angry and rebellious feelings. Often when an adolescent has AN, peer relationships have either failed to develop or have been abandoned due to the psychological or physical sequelae of the illness. The intense focus required to maintain the disorder often make the adolescent so preoccupied that she becomes uninterested or is perceived to be uninterested in her peers. On the other hand, the severe malnutrition also leads to problems with energy and attention and sometimes to physical health problems that require hospitalization. These, too, have a negative impact on peer relationships. Therefore, as the adolescent with AN begins to recover, she may discover she has lost ground in this area, and she may require therapeutic assistance to rekindle her relationships. Because of the illness and its treatment, parents and family members may be more reluctant to support these peer relationships. Families need help in "letting go" of their daughter sufficiently so they can support her developing need for relationships outside the home.

Some older adolescents may be entering the late stage of adolescence as they complete treatment. For them, relevant issues are principally those that involve planning for college and careers and practicing for deeper interpersonal relationships outside the family. In general, this stage is characterized by the increasing wish and ability for emotional and sexual intimacy and less need for support from the family. Problems that might arise in this phase are derived from residual problems in these areas, such as continued excessive emotional or physical dependency on parents or family, continued anxiety about sexual abilities or body image, and anxiety about the meaning of personal intimacy in terms of procreation. All of these issues can be adversely affected by AN. Studies have suggested that even with recovery from the physical aspects of AN, interpersonal difficulties often remain. In addition, because the adolescent with AN has been more dependent on her parents for emotional and physical support, attachment to figures outside the home has been delayed. This may be especially true for romantic and sexual partners. In addition, the adolescent with AN may be especially reluctant to share her body with another because of her fears about the acceptability of her body shape. The adolescent with AN has also had to manage the real possibility of infertility because of the lack of menses that characterizes the disorder. Family therapy is especially important in helping the family, who may be anxious about supporting the development of romantic relationships or who may prevent the exploration of career or educational opportunities that take the adolescent from home.

Parents, too, must accomplish developmental tasks associated with the process of adolescence in their children. Following are some suggestions that may help parents during this transitional phase of treatment:

- Develop activities, interests, and skills that constitute a post-parenting life.
- Develop an identity as a couple.
- Discover ways in which parental roles, work, leisure interests, and studies can be integrated with the interests and needs of the developing adults in the household.
- Accept the distinctive physical and emotional aspects of the sexual development, orientation, and interests of growing adolescents.
- Give up the skills, attitudes, and activities that were appropriate to earlier developmental stages of children.
- Evolve personal capacities that increase adolescents' ability to see and accept parents as developing individuals.

Each of these topics may become a theme in Phase III of treatment. The failure of parents to accomplish these tasks may make it more difficult for the adolescent to complete her own transition to adulthood. Therapists may use this list as a way to help identify a specific focus for the interventions with the couple that are used during this treatment phase.

Teamwork in Phase III

Teamwork will likely have evolved from Phase I to Phase III, with decreasing intensity of involvement with the team members who are outside the direct therapeutic intervention. Often, by the time a patient reaches Phase III, nutritionists and pediatricians have decreased their monitoring of the patient, as the patient's documented progress makes it safe for them to do so. However, it is likely that the patient will continue to maintain these relationships at least until the conclusion of therapy, and she should be encouraged to do so. These visits, like the therapy sessions, are likely to be spaced at greater and greater time intervals.

The relationship among the therapeutic team itself (e.g., cotherapists) remains as active and as important as ever. As the family moves toward termination, they may attempt to involve one or both of the therapists in family dynamics as a way of undermining this process. Termination may also be difficult for therapists who have invested in the recovery of this patient and family. The therapeutic team can help identify these issues more clearly so that they can be approached systematically.

Reviewing Adolescent Issues with the Family and Modeling Problem Solving of These Types of Issues

Why

Because many adolescents with AN develop problems in negotiating general adolescent developmental issues, it is important to assist the patient and family in re-integrating the patient into adolescence after the episode of AN has subsided. This is true because the illness itself often requires the adolescent to be absent from school and to remain dependent on her parents because of her medical and psychological needs for help with refeeding. In this way, she may be out of sync with her peers. Upon successful weight restoration and adequate self-feeding, these other issues may need to be addressed. It is expected that there may be a large range of needs in this area, depending on the resources that both the individual patient and the family have to bring to bear on the problems. For example, in a relatively uncomplicated case in which refeeding is achieved with little difficulty and in which few other types of family problems exist, getting the adolescent back on track may be fairly straightforward. On the other hand, when the refeeding process in Phases I and II does not proceed so smoothly or is complicated by other family or individual problems, more work may be required in Phase III. In Phase III, the patient's anger about how she has been treated during the refeeding process may become a focus. It is helpful for parents to acknowledge what they can of the daughter's complaints about what has been taken from her.

It must be emphasized that the approach described here is more applicable to relatively uncomplicated cases. A separate course of adolescent family psychotherapy may well be required in more complicated cases, and the issues that need to be addressed may go well beyond the outlines provided in this manual.

How

It may be necessary for the therapist to begin this phase by reviewing the progress the patient and family have made together thus far. In this way, the pertinent themes that the therapist identified in the earlier sessions and that were deferred in order to address the distorted eating behavior can be brought to light. The primer on adolescent issues and AN provided herein can serve as a template for the therapist in providing this review. We suggest that the therapist begin by being prepared to give a kind of "mini-lecture" on adolescent development, using the three-stage model described previously. This technique allows the therapist to identify a range of themes for the family to consider. It also helps to ensure that most relevant themes are included. More emotionally charged issues, such as sexual development and behavior, might need special emphasis, as the family might otherwise attempt to avoid these. This review should take no more than 10 minutes.

Involving the Family in "Review" of Issues

Why

Involving the family in the review of adolescent issues as related to their own adolescent's development helps the family to identify and specify areas of concern. It also helps to reinforce the minilecture on adolescent development through some repetition and by making the information more personally relevant.

How

As discussed at the end of Phase II, the therapist and family can now address some of the identified issues of adolescence. For example, the therapist might mention that, early in the therapy, the patient complained about how her mother interfered with her choice of friends and then ask the patient to elaborate on this issue. It is helpful if the therapist is able to identify issues raised by all family members. (This process requires that the therapist be alert to and keep a record of Phase III issues from the outset of the therapeutic interventions. It might help to make note of these so they can be used as concrete examples when the time comes in Phase III.) It is important that the therapist help to enable the family to solve the problems of adolescent development that confront them. This is akin to the strategy employed in Phase I of empowering the family to deal with AN. The aim here is to engage the family in the process of adolescence and to authorize them to approach and deal with the problems that are involved as they apply to their own family.

After a set of these key issues are identified, the therapist may find it helpful to spend a few minutes providing an overview of the process of adolescence and the types of issues that all families with teenagers are likely to encounter. This will help to educate the patient and family about the process of adolescence and help them see it as normal.

Next, the therapist should attempt to integrate the issues identified by the patient and family into the overall scheme of adolescent development. This process should actively involve the family. The therapist should provide guidance in this process but not take it over.

Delineating and Exploring Adolescent Themes

Why

In order to assist the family in finding ways to manage the adolescent process now that the eating-disordered behavior is behind them, the therapist may provide targeted assistance in problem solving that may serve as a template for their efforts at home after completion of therapy. It is important for the family to explore some of the issues of adolescence without the eating problems interfering or becoming the idiom of this process. The family should be confident that they have other capacities to manage issues now that the eating disorder is no longer present.

How

The therapist can use the "circular" questioning strategy employed in earlier sessions. This technique involves the whole family and helps to "flesh" out the issues. Sufficient detail about the problem must be evident to allow the therapist to provide the family with material for interpretation. By this point, of course, the therapist has a sophisticated understanding of how this family is likely to approach (or not approach) problems. This is a considerable advantage, as the way the family managed the problem with eating and weight is likely to be similar to how it may manage other problems of adolescence. For example, if the theme is the need to support the development of peer friendships for the adolescent with AN, the therapist might begin by asking each parent about his or her view of the importance of friends; next, the therapist asks if the adolescent agrees with this and if she feels supported by her family in developing friendships. If there are other adolescent family members, their views should also be solicited. As the family describes their thoughts and experience, the therapist should be preparing to provide assistance where there are problems. If, for example, it is clear that the parents are overly restrictive, the therapist may ask the family why this is so and what would make them more open to friendships. A dialogue should ensue that allows the therapist, patient, and family to come to an agreement about how best to make friendships more available within the context of the parent's concerns.

Checking How Much the Parents Are Doing as a Couple

Why

Parents must also successfully negotiate their own relationship after the immediate crisis of the eating disorder has passed. Much of the therapy has encouraged joint parental action in the face of the difficulties of refeeding their daughter. This may have become the main way in which the couple has related to each other for some time. However, at this point, in order to support the increased appropriate autonomy of their daughter and to support their own relationship, focusing on the parents' needs for a relationship is warranted.

It may seem that little is likely to be accomplished with such an intervention. This may indeed be true if there are major relationship problems. However, in many cases, the eating disorder and its treatment are the source of any derailment in the parental dyad. In these cases, simply indicating that there is a potential problem that may need to be addressed is sufficient to set things on the right course. On the other hand, parental difficulties that predate the eating disorder may have been put aside in the interest of their daughter's health. These problems may reemerge at this juncture, but the therapy outlined here is unlikely to address these types of problems. Instead, the couple may seek additional treatment elsewhere.

How

This therapy is not an attempt at an abbreviated couples therapy, any more than it is an attempt to complete a full-fledged family therapy for emerging adolescents. Instead, the idea is to identify the need for the couple to consider their own relationship in the changed context of their daughter's renewed health and entry into adolescence. In order to get the couple to accomplish this, the therapist asks them how much time they spend together, what they do, and how these answers compare with their past experiences of one another. The therapist does not need to intervene with specific ideas about how to improve the relationship's structure but instead encourages the couple to explore these issues.

Planning for Future Issues

Why

It is important to support the family by indicating ways they might proceed in the future. This helps to communicate both the therapist's continuing investment in the family and some specific ways to proceed if problems occur.

How

The therapist can assist in this task by providing some guidance about what kinds of issues the future might hold, such as the patient leaving for college or work, by suggesting different ways the family might approach problems, by raising targeted issues that could not be explored previously, and so forth. Again the therapist should be alert to the time and emphasis placed on this therapeutic maneuver. It is important that all family members have an opportunity to participate and be involved in this discussion. It is also likely that the patient's and parents' issues may dominate the discussion, but this should be less evident than in the previous maneuver.

Terminating Treatment

Why

As important as greeting the family at the onset of treatment is the process of respectfully bidding adieu. This process should clearly end the therapeutic relationship by conferring on the family the sincere confidence that they can proceed with likely success if future problems arise. The treatment for AN using the family model described in this book lasts approximately 1 year. Although the early interventions are the most intense and most closely spaced, the involvement with the family is significant over this period. The early use of the therapist's authority to impress on the family the seriousness of the illness, as well as the use of paradoxical interventions throughout the therapy, make the relationship with the therapist that much more intense. Over Phases II and III, great effort is made to decrease the dependence on the therapist while also increasing both the patient's and the family's autonomous functioning in line with the ultimate goal of a successful termination. The method of termination employed here is one of many that could be used. The key concern is that the family has an opportunity to review the therapy and say good-bye to the therapist, whereas the therapist has an opportunity to lend the family optimism and support in the process of separation.

How

The therapist should reserve part of the last session to conclude the therapy by saying good-bye to each family member. This process should mirror the momentous and careful greeting of each family member that took place in Session 1. The therapist should pay attention to each family member's involvement, praise each one for his or her work commitment on behalf of the family, and maintain a demeanor of genuine warmth, comfort, and subdued optimism. Family members should each be given an opportunity to bid the therapist farewell. The therapist's aim is to encourage the family's abilities to proceed smoothly and undertake successfully any problems that are ahead.

The principal method in this session is listening. The therapist asks each family member in turn to review his or her experience of the therapy from start to finish. The emphasis is on each family member and on the family as a whole to prepare for ending the therapeutic relationship. The therapist may help this process along by demarcating the phases of the therapy and emphasizing certain issues that arose for each family member in the process. The process should begin with the parents, followed by the patient and siblings. Care should be taken to include all family members, though, by necessity, more time is likely to be taken up by the parents and the patient. The therapist must carefully time this session, as no more that about one-half the allotted time is used for this "reminiscing."

Common Questions about Phase III

What if the family persists in using food and weight concerns in adolescent–parent communication?

It may be that in some families, even though the worst symptoms of weight loss and concern have passed, there is a persistent pattern of using weight and food concerns as a way of communicating with one another. In these cases, the therapist's aim should be to identify the reasons that this focus remains. Other concerns about adolescence may help to refocus the family on more appropriate issues. The therapist may find it helpful to directly explore the food and weight preoccupations of the family as a whole at this juncture to gain a better understanding of such a continued focus.

What if the family denies that there are other adolescent issues or problems?

Some families find it difficult to see issues or problems that may be present in their families. It is important not to "make problems" for such families. Instead, the therapist may want to use the strategy of a general review that is provided to discuss the typical issues associated with adolescents. This way, any issues can be identified in a nonpathological manner, and discussion can occur in way that is noncritical of the family.

What if the family is not involved in the review of adolescent process review?

One of the possible problems associated with this therapeutic maneuver is that the therapist can become a "lecturer" on adolescence.

Although the therapist should be seen as an expert guide to the adolescent process, the review should be collaborative and should provide opportunities for interaction with family members.

What if the parents do not feel that they should spend time with each other separately from the family?

Rarely, couples believe that they do not need time together apart from their children. This may be particularly true in families in which the patient is an only child. In such cases, it is helpful to remind the parents that soon their daughter will be leaving home and that it may be good practice for them and for her to do things separately from each other.

13

Phase III in Action

*I*n this chapter, we provide an example of a session near the completion of Phase III. The therapist reviews adolescent issues and prepares for termination.

Clinical Background

This is the same family whose therapy experiences are detailed in Session 2 (Chapter 7) and Phase II (Chapter 11). The patient has progressed well, has resumed normal eating on her own, and has maintained a healthy weight long enough to achieve a return of menses. The family is understandably pleased with her progress and feel prepared to conclude treatment.

To review, the major goals for Phase III of treatment are:

- To establish that the adolescent–parent relationship no longer requires the symptoms as an idiom of communication.
- To review adolescent issues with the family and to model problem solving of these types of issues
- To terminate treatment.

In order to accomplish these goals, the therapist undertakes the following interventions:

1. Reviewing adolescent issues with the family and modeling problem solving of these types of issues.
2. Involving the family in "review" of issues.
3. Checking how much the parents are doing as a couple.
4. Delineating and exploring adolescent themes.
5. Planning for future issues.
6. Terminating treatment.

THERAPIST: All right, how did it go last week?

RHONDA: Well, I remember what I told you, and I was trying to get there, but I wasn't comfortable with going faster. I was comfortable with having a little bit more, but not a whole lot more. But I was comfortable with what I was doing, and I'm doing really well. So I didn't want to do something that I gain weight and then lose it, so. . . .

THERAPIST: So it's been a steady climb.

RHONDA: And if I have a weight gain next week, I can go to the pediatrician only once every other week. So they're happy with what I've been doing.

THERAPIST: So have they started talking to you about exercising?

RHONDA: They just ask me, "Do you exercise?" But my form of exercise would be riding, so, I mean, they don't want me riding. Basically in so many words, they don't come out and tell me, but that was basically what they say.

THERAPIST: Have you asked them when that would be okay?

RHONDA: Well, right now, unfortunately, where I board my horse, she had her house for sale for awhile, but she's moving. So I'm in the process of thinking of moving him, but I'm moving him to a place where I can ride. But I have the option of riding in the ring, which will be more time, or riding on a trail, which would be less time. Which I don't know. There is a ring down below, that the guy that owns the ring said we can use the ring, but I don't want to ask because I don't know him. So I wouldn't ask. So that's okay.

THERAPIST: So have you asked your pediatrician what you will need to weigh for them to let you ride?

RHONDA: It's more of a bone thing, but that's not until January, so if I feel good. . . .

THERAPIST: Do you think that they would let you, since you have a return of your menses?

RHONDA: But, they said that they can't say exactly when, even if, I'll keep it, even if I'm at my target weight. They said it's different for everybody. You might not get it again until a couple months later.

THERAPIST: It's true, we talked about this, there is no magic formula. People can give you numbers, but what your body tells you is a better indication. But you have a rough idea of what it is, because you already had menses before, so your body is not likely to have changed. It may take a little while to kick in, that's true. Sometimes your body wants to make sure, before it wastes any energy.

RHONDA: I remember you saying that last time.

THERAPIST: I guess I'm encouraging you to think about asking them how they are going to work this thing out. Say, "Okay, look."

In the preceding series of questions and interventions, the therapist engages Rhonda in a dialogue about her interest in making further progress so that she can exercise regularly, in this case by riding her horse. The therapist aims to increase Rhonda's investment in making progress on her own. This is distinguished from similar strategies directed toward the parents in earlier sessions. At this point, the therapist considers the eating and weight concerns largely in Rhonda's hands and wants to reinforce this. The therapist also asks that Rhonda take active interest in finding out information about her current health from her pediatrician to reinforce her more autonomous development.

RHONDA: Well, going every other week is a good start.

THERAPIST: It's a good start, you feel, you feel better about it. (*to parents*) How about the two of you? How do you think she is doing?

MOTHER: I think she's doing really well.

FATHER: Yeah, very good.

MOTHER: And, we're backing off a lot, so she is more independent now as far as her goals.

RHONDA: He's not talking about my goals, Mom, he's talking about eating.

MOTHER: But I meant goals as far as getting back into the normalcy of eating.

THERAPIST: And what have the two of you done to back off? You sort of moved a little bit away but not too far last time. You let her serve herself. . . .

FATHER: It's completely in her hands now.

THERAPIST: Completely?

FATHER: Yeah, we don't even ask Rhonda . . . Well, that's not true, I do ask what she had for lunch. I see what she eats for breakfast, and we know what she eats for dinner.

MOTHER: We'll ask her, "What did you have, or where did you go for lunch?"

FATHER: Yeah, "Where did you go."

MOTHER: We'll ask her that way, and she'll say, "Well, I went to La Boulangerie, and I had a salad, or a turkey sandwich."

FATHER: But we're not doing that to check up on her, it's just inquisitive, because I know she's eating really well.

THERAPIST: And so, so you two from that perspective have really given up monitoring her food and weight. (*to Rhonda*) Do you feel that difference?

RHONDA: It's the same as before to me, it's the same as before.

THERAPIST: So you feel like you were doing it on your own before, and now you're doing it on your own still?

RHONDA: Pretty much, pretty much. I mean it's up to me how I'm doing. Because if I'm with my friends or something, I have to choose what I'm going to eat then anyway.

In the preceding series of interventions, the therapist engages the parents as a couple directly, distinct from the previous maneuver, which was directed at Rhonda exclusively. The aim for the therapist is to continue to support the parental dyad specifically in the context of their management together of the process of "backing off" from the monitoring of Rhonda's food intake and weight.

Reviewing Adolescent Issues with the Family and Modeling Problem Solving of These Types of Issues

THERAPIST: So everybody is feeling more independent around all of these things in a sense. Well, that sort of tells us, tells me, that we're definitely in a period of wrapping up the focus on the eating part and are working on whatever issues about adolescence that may be a part of your family that you want to explore, get some idea about. How you might have affected your adolescence by getting this disorder, how you might keep it from recurring. I wondered if you might have any thoughts on that?

RHONDA: Like as far as, like, what are you asking?

THERAPIST: At the beginning of therapy, I said that sessions we have toward the end would be about general issues in adolescence, and maybe how eating affected them, and maybe see if there was a connection to your problem with developing anorexia. You know we really didn't talk about any of that, instead, we went right in, and that's the way this particular therapy works. Now you're healthy enough to really think about those things, if they are still there. And, you know, adolescence is a two-way street in a sense that you (*to the parents*) are in adolescence with her. Being parents of an adolescent is very different from all the other times of being a parent. You may need to parent differently, and your lives are affected differently as a result of adolescence, as compared to newborns or school-age children. And one of the things you had to do right away is probably something you never thought you'd have to do. Deal with anorexia. . . .

FATHER: We never really thought of it, although we did give it thought as we would see movies or read articles in the paper, maybe hear of an athlete that was diagnosed with it, and we would think about it as, "Gee, that's terrible." Like everybody says that first we ever heard about it was with the singer, Karen Carpenter, and gave it a lot of thought because I had actually seen her on television very close to the end of her life, and she was singing and she still had a magnificent voice. When I looked at her and she came out I almost died, because I said, "Oh my God," she looked like she was skin and bones. Because her face, you actually could see her skull, because her skin pulled in to her eyes, and it was really very scary. And she died shortly after that, and when I heard she had died from that, I said I knew something was wrong with her. How anyone could think they looked good . . . or maybe it wasn't that she thought she looked good, it could have been just sickness that got a hold of her, because she battled that for years, from what I understand.

MOTHER: From what I hear, from other people recovering or trying to get over this disease, Rhonda has gone through in very little time, as compared to other people. It would take 10 years or 7 to 8 years or something, you know. It just started just after her senior year started. Everyone I talked to said it's going to be a long, drawn-out process, it's going to be years, and I see how Rhonda is progressing, it's less than a year.

FATHER: Rhonda is very strong, too, if she puts her mind to something she can do it.

THERAPIST: What do you think about all this?

RHONDA: Well, that's true, if I want something bad enough, I'll get it. You know what may have happened, too, when I was thinking back. After the summer when I was with my friends a lot, you know, I wasn't eating right, but I never thought about it, but I wasn't eating right. Because we were doing things, we might have gone to the movies or something, I just wasn't, like, eating what I was supposed to. And when I went back to school, I got compliments and stuff, that I lost a little bit of weight, and then some teachers were saying, "I hope you're not fading away on us." And I was still like 105 pounds and I was, like, "Oh, this is nice." So I just started. . . .

THERAPIST: Why do you think you liked it?

RHONDA: I don't know, it was nice to be complimented about it.

THERAPIST: It's a big thing in the world of women in general, huh?

MOTHER: The image you project.

THERAPIST: Well, this whole weight loss thing, it's a big part of women's culture to always be asking, you know, "Well, did you lose weight? Are you on a diet? Or, what kind of diet are you on?" And being strong minded, it's easier for someone who is strong minded to be very successful at dieting. It's sometimes how this whole thing gets started. Because they are determined and have a specific goal. It's also a very precise kind of goal, . . . to lose weight, it's not vague at all. Compared to some of the other things in adolescence that you might be up against, it's kind of easy. Like, you know, some things that are tough in adolescence are dealing with . . . that's why I asked why. . . .

RHONDA: Because you were thinking what boys thought of me? Is that it?

THERAPIST: Not exactly, though that's interesting, too, but I was thinking more about how you thought of yourself. But sometimes that figures into it too, how other people think about you affects how you think about yourself, that often includes boys in high school.

RHONDA: Well, I never thought, "Oh, God, I hope they think I look okay." And stuff like that. Because I really didn't care, you know, I was happy, I had my friends and my friends didn't care. So I really didn't, either, if they like me, they like me, if they don't, they don't. You are always going to go through life, and some people may not like you because of the way you look and some may not like you because they don't like your personality. My school is very much on fashion and stuff in a way . . . not so much how you look but the clothes you wear. But everyone has their own style. But they are still, like, "Oh, my God, what's that one wearing?" But I don't pay attention to that, because if you do pay attention to that type of stuff, where people are judging you, you are going to go through life feeling maybe a little paranoid.

THERAPIST: I couldn't agree with that more, that's great. But what I was talking about was sort of the general challenge of adolescence. There are three big things that happen in adolescence that are different, that are different from being sort of a school-age child in a lot of ways, or being preschool, or whatever. One is your body changes a lot, that starts at 11, 12, 13, usually, and that's a big adjustment. You know, you get taller, your body develops a sexual shape, and suddenly your body is not what you were thinking about before, it's radically different. It's the biggest physical change that you go through, really, in life, in one fell swoop. Umm, other than the first 12 months of your life, there is just so much going on physically. So, there's that. So that's one big adjustment. Another big adjustment is you have social independence, just as you were describing. You and your friends. In a way that, maybe your parents have heard some of it, but they don't know all of it, they can't see it all the time. Before, in grade school, there was some of that, it is really a whole lot harder to see everything in these years than it was before. And so that whole area, developing a sort of social identity, is very challenging, too. Now, now it is a little bit different because you are farther outside the family. And the third thing, which is something we've talked about, is just thinking about work, your future in terms of career, what you want to be. So all of those three things are big tasks for an adolescent, and every one is a parallel task for a parent. For parents, having their child develop an adolescent body can be very challenging, they are not prepared for it often. It can be as exciting as having your child take their first steps, but it can also be kind of "Oh my gosh, there I have a grown person." It's very different. Second, social issues bring up all sorts of things with families. Things like, Do I like their friends? Are they good friends? Are they not so good friends? Who is she liking? Will sex be involved? When will that start? All those kinds of questions. And then of course with career and with choices about life. You (*to the parents*) have dreams and wishes for your child often, and whether spoken or unspoken, they make a difference in terms of this process of learning.

FATHER: Everybody goes through it.

THERAPIST: That's right.

RHONDA: And I'm not looking forward to going through it with my kids.

FATHER: But everybody goes through it, and most people fare very well.

THERAPIST: That's really true, you know, they used to talk about in studies of adolescence as a troubled time, actually most adolescents do very well. I mean, they do a little bit of stuff, and everybody does a little bit of stuff, but they overall turn out pretty solid.

RHONDA: I have to agree with you, even though a lot of people are not too sure of what they are going to do, or sometimes they have problems with some friends or other friends, they overall do good. As far as coping with . . . if they have problems, but overall they do good.

FATHER: That's all in the upbringing, too, from day 1 at birth, I think.

The therapist attempts to involve the family in an initial review of common issues for adolescents and their parents. In this case, the family does not feel that there are problems of this sort in their family. The therapist respects this but provides the information about possible issues to allow a nonpathological way of discussing adolescent development.

Involving the Family in "Review" of Issues

THERAPIST: But thinking about those three kinds of major themes, where, do you think, (*to parents*) let's start with the two of you. Rhonda has kind of given us a little preview of who she is, so let's start with the two of you. Where do you think you are and Rhonda is on those three points, those three major areas there, sort of outlines, tasks of adolescence.

FATHER: Well, as far as her developing into adolescence, I don't understand how some people could be bothered by it. Really, I never would even give it a second thought. Because from birth, in raising Rhonda, from day 1 until right now, we look at it as being very normal. And I have always been one person to, as far as a person's weight, never to hold, if I like a person, I like a person's personality, that's most important to me. It doesn't have anything to do with money, weight. And I think Rhonda knows this, and I think she's pretty much the same way, too. As far as her education is concerned, that's strictly up to Rhonda, and I think Rhonda is going in the right direction.

THERAPIST: That's a good thing.

FATHER: What was the other thing?

MOTHER: Her friends.

FATHER: Honestly, I have been very comfortable with Rhonda's friends.

MOTHER: For the most part.

FATHER: Yeah, almost 95% of them are very polite, and nice kids, good kids. Because first of all I don't think Rhonda would go around with a crowd. And I can sympathize with parents, you hear these horror stories, your kids got into the wrong group, then how do they control them? You know sometimes it's too late. I think that's the upbringing really. Children know right from wrong. Just like adults do.

RHONDA: Well, they can also. When you go into high school, and you're looking for a group of friends . . . It's the type of person you are. If you're kind of insecure about yourself, and you're afraid that people won't accept you, and the first group of people that come up to you, whether they are a good group or they have a bad influence on you, if you are insecure about yourself, you will just go in with that group. But if you actually think about it, and you have opinions about the friends you want to hang out with, not limiting it to a certain type of group, but just saying that, you know, I don't want to hang out with people that have drugs as their life, I mean I have friends that have done drugs, they don't influence me, though. My friends mostly don't smoke, don't do drugs, don't drink alcohol, most of them, but some of them do. But they don't care if you do it or not, they just care that it's their choice. But I've never been confronted. I was scared of this in junior high, because they said, you're going to be confronted, people are going to say, "Here, smoke this, or drink this, or take this." I haven't been. I don't know if it's maybe the area I live in, too. But I haven't been confronted, they mostly, you know, if you want to do something, it's your choice, but they make their own choice to do that. I've never felt pressured into doing anything, and I would never put myself in that situation, too, personally.

THERAPIST: *(to the mother)* What about you? What are your perspectives on these three major tasks?

FATHER: He put her on the spot *(smiling)*.

THERAPIST: What do you mean?

FATHER: Because you're always joking.

MOTHER: I was saying, about the social issue, in the early stages of her disease, I noticed that she was alienating herself from her friends. Whereas, like last summer, if we got to see her at dinner, we were lucky. And when she was home she was on the phone for 3, 4 hours. But then when she started getting sick and was really going through this thing in the beginning, she was seeing less and less of her friends, talking less. And then she kept saying, "Well, all my friends are immature." And she wanted to go to [College Y] at one point, because all of her friends were going. Now she wants to go to a completely different junior college, so no one else is going, so she can make a new set of friends and start a whole new life and everything. And I really commend her for that, I really do.

FATHER: A lot of people say that, too, when you tell them.

MOTHER: I know, and they all say, "I think that's a really wise decision." Because if Rhonda went to [College Y], all of her friends would be, like high school, in the same clique and everything. But now, she wants to grow up.

RHONDA: But my main friends are mostly going away to state colleges or universities. Like my best friend, she's going to X State, so she's going away. But a lot of people that I know, that I just talk to, you know, just small talk, they're going to another college. I'd say most, not most, maybe a quarter to half the senior class, they're going to [X]. About all of them are. It's quite a high number. But I like [College Y]. I was very impressed with them, because, remember, I told you, I went to that day, where you sign up for your classes, orientation, and they had the counselors there so you could sign up for your classes, and print your schedule, and get the bill that same day. Well, [College X], I don't know what they were doing, but they said they would have counselors there, and they never showed up. All these kids had to reschedule signing up for class. And they stalled by doing a longer orientation. I wasn't impressed with what I heard from them. And they also do another thing called the "smart system" where you call and you sign up by phone, and that can be confusing, too. And I don't believe [College Y] does that, I don't think.

THERAPIST: What's going on with the other tasks?

MOTHER: Physically, her development, umm. I have always thought as she's been growing up, she's developed very well. She was slow in every type of stage, you know, she was slow in lifting her head up, potty training, walking, talking, but my maternal grandmother always said, "It's not when she starts, it's the end result." So with that kind of attitude, I really didn't care if she was late or what. And here she is, she's a beautiful young woman. And the only thing I was disappointed in was that, when she stopped her period, that kind of put a roadblock, kind of detoured a little. But I think once her body gets used to eating well now, I think that will start up. And I think this whole thing probably taught Rhonda a lesson about eating well nutritionally, not so much watching what she eats or how she eats, but just making sure she eats well and enough, and that's all she needs, and I think she's learned that.

THERAPIST: So from your perspective, when she entered puberty, it didn't create any new problems for her?

MOTHER: No.

THERAPIST: How about work and career? What are your thoughts on what Rhonda will do with her life?

MOTHER: Well, she has lots of interests, at one point she maybe wanted to have a catering business because she liked to cook. But I think it was because you were doing so much cooking and everything.

RHONDA: Yeah, I remember that.

MOTHER: Because I think you wanted to cook a lot, but you never ate it, you always pawned it off on me and Dad.

RHONDA: Yeah, whether it was a disaster or not.

MOTHER: At one point you wanted to be a vet a long time ago, then you said you didn't want to operate, or do any operation.

RHONDA: Right, but I found out, it's not . . . What bothers me is operating on humans. I couldn't do that, I could never do that. Whether it's being naive or not, I don't want to see what I look like inside. It's just too close to, I guess you could say, home. But animals wouldn't bother me. Large animals, I think, for the most part.

MOTHER: I always wanted her to have a good education, I pretty much was the one that would always help her with her homework. I even say that now, "Do you have any homework?"

THERAPIST: Habits are hard to break.

RHONDA: I've gotten better in my spelling. I remember at grade school, when they go to look over my essay, they would laugh, in the kitchen. I would laugh, because I knew I spelled a lot of words wrong. I even laughed before I gave it to them, because I knew that I spelled a lot of words wrong because I was terrible at spelling. But I got better, thank God, because I don't think my English teacher in college would like it if I spelled wrong.

THERAPIST: Do you have Spell Check?

RHONDA: Well, yeah, but then sometimes it's also grammar.

MOTHER: They don't have grammar checks in the computer.

RHONDA: Yeah, they do.

The therapist proceeds to try to involve the family as a whole in the review of adolescent issues. The therapist carefully reviews each major theme with all three family members in this case, as what may be an issue with one family member may not be with another. The tone of the inquiry is one of interest and aims to engage all members in thinking about these issues.

Delineating and Exploring Adolescent Themes

THERAPIST: Well, let me throw some challenges out, well, not challenges, thoughts about what you've said, and some things that I would like to see what more you think about. First of all, the image you painted of Rhonda last summer, before anorexia really took over, what did you say, "Lucky if you saw her at dinner, and when she was home she was always on the phone." And then you said, "Well, and then it all went away," kind of like she was maybe before she was a teenager, or eating with you all the time, more being there, in your presence all the time, at home. She wasn't out there, in the way that she was. What's normal in adolescence is exactly what you said, the picture of Rhonda being social and active and so forth, and so encouraging that part, to the degree, there is also a little sense, I have to say in your tone, a little sadness, and a little loss, "Where was she?" Every parent should feel a little like that.

MOTHER: Well, I was always worried when she wasn't home yet and it got dark.

THERAPIST: Yeah, but didn't you miss her?

MOTHER: Of course I did.

THERAPIST: It's sometimes hard, because they're focused on your world. Not that you don't have your own things to do, but you're used to her being there. So that's enough of what I wanted to add, sort of see if you can remember that a little bit.

FATHER: When she gets married, she's going to be gone.

RHONDA: Except when I find a spider.

FATHER: Yeah, then she'll call us.

MOTHER: Yeah, in the middle of the night. A little tiny spider and she goes hysterical. I said, "Well, if you had your own place, and you're married, are you going to call us up to come over there?"

THERAPIST: The answer is yes?

RHONDA: I freak out, I can't stand bugs, and that's kind of strange because I ride horses all the time, but when you're preoccupied with something, you know, and when you're with the horse, it's an open area, so you don't see all the little bugs.

MOTHER: You know, when I was concerned about, in the summertime when she was gone a lot during the day, I would be concerned if she got home on time, but then when she was home . . . I think I lost my train of thought.

THERAPIST: That's okay, we'll wait. We were talking about how it felt last summer, sometimes you'd worry that she wouldn't be home on time.

RHONDA: Driving in the dark.

FATHER: Oh, yeah, that concerned me because she was just starting to drive. Plus with all those idiots on the road.

THERAPIST: That's a good example, too, you've been driving her, now she's behind the wheel, too, and not just her, it's everybody.

FATHER: Because she's a good driver.

MOTHER: But then when she's home, a lot of times I would get angry with her when she was on the phone, because I said, "Well, what if someone needs to get a hold of us." And she'd get after us, "Well, get call waiting." But who is that going to benefit?

THERAPIST: So those kinds of issues you struggled with, and then found ways to work on them.

MOTHER: Oh, yeah.

THERAPIST: That's great. So let me throw out another one for you, how about dating and sex? How is that one handled?

RHONDA: I've only had two boyfriends.

THERAPIST: Did your parents meet them?

RHONDA: Yeah, you met both of them.

FATHER: Tom and Tony.

RHONDA: That was my sophomore year, and he was a freshman. That lasted all of a month. And Tom was Laura's, my best friend's, brother.

MOTHER: Is.

RHONDA: Is, sorry.

THERAPIST: Was your boyfriend, still is?

RHONDA: Still is her brother. I don't know, maybe I just can't have a long relationship. But he was jealous of his sister, because I was always with his sister and I would always talk to her on the phone, and he thought I should be talking to him on the phone, not his sister. But I said to him, because its always the case where, your friends come before. If you have a boyfriend, your friends come before them, no matter what, that's how it should be, the same with guys, but it's usually not. I don't know, then he got jealous, and all the time I was with him, I was fighting with him in some ways.

MOTHER: But you guys are still good friends.

RHONDA: Yeah, he's still nice, he's still nice, I don't hold any grudges or anything.

FATHER: Jealousy is a form of sickness, as far as I'm concerned. It's not normal and it's not right. But everybody is different.

THERAPIST: So what did you think about these boyfriends? It was some new territory for you, too.

FATHER: I didn't know Tony that well, Tom. . . .

THERAPIST: Apparently not, you put him out of your mind?

FATHER: Tom I do know, very polite young man, very polite. I didn't have a problem with that as long as I knew where they were going. And then of course Rhonda did . . . I don't know if it was her fault or not. The time they were going to a movie and dinner, and they ended up at the beach. That I didn't particularly care for. Tell the truth, because in case of an accident or something should happen . . . That's the only reason.

RHONDA: I didn't know that. And he was like, "Now I'm afraid, because I was taking you to Santa Cruz to surprise you, and now I'm afraid because your parents are mad at me."

FATHER: Well, I did say don't ever do it again.

RHONDA: Well, I didn't know, it wasn't my fault.

THERAPIST: So a different kind of vigilance gets aroused around having a boyfriend in the whole mix, right? You're worried about where he's going to take her, and yet it's also a private world for you, it's your own private domain. I mean, he's your boyfriend. He still has to have some relationship with you. How about you, how was, do you remember Tony?

MOTHER: I just met him one time, when we dropped Rhonda off at a dance.

FATHER: I do remember I liked him.

MOTHER: And then he broke it off, for one reason or another, and she got upset about that. And, but I think she got over it real quick, but just the initial. . . .

RHONDA: No, he didn't. We were talking and I don't know what he was . . . because he was a freshman, and. . . .

THERAPIST: You were at that time, a sophomore?

RHONDA: Sophomore. But I don't know, but I was just saying to him, "Well, I don't think it's working out." And he was like, "So what do you want to do?" And I was like, "I don't think we should be together." And he was like, "That's what I think." So it was like a mutual thing.

THERAPIST: What did you think about Bobby?

MOTHER: Bobby is a very nice young man.

THERAPIST: What do you think about the whole process of Rhonda starting to date?

MOTHER: Well, she hasn't really started . . . I think she is pretty consumed with her horse and her girlfriends.

RHONDA: I haven't, the last person I talked to was Andy, and he's the one who brought me in to the counselor. He brought me in to the counselor, because he thought I had a problem.

THERAPIST: Andy is a boyfriend?

RHONDA: But he was just a friend, though, but he brought me into the counselor because he said, the more he was talking to me and everything, he thought I had a problem. And he was one of my friend's . . . well, she wasn't my friend, she was my friend's friend. I just knew her through that. That was her brother. And he went to [Z school]. And he thought I had a problem.

MOTHER: And he met you one day?

RHONDA: Yeah, to bring me to the counselor, because he didn't believe me that I go and talk to them about it. He was nice, but . . . And I had no reason to stop talking to him, but I just, because I went into the hospital, and then when I came out, he still called, but I just never talked to him. I just didn't talk to him since I went into the hospital.

THERAPIST: But that was the last boy you were sort of interested in?

RHONDA: Umm, yeah, he was nice.

FATHER: No, Bobby was.

RHONDA: Bobby was in July.

THERAPIST: Boyfriends go by the month?

RHONDA: No, not to make it sound like that, but that was in July.

MOTHER: This was after senior year started.

RHONDA: I mean he was nice, just kind of not my type.

Here the therapist tries to examine the issues more deeply with the family. From the earlier "review" and "discussion," the therapist identifies a number of possible areas in which problems might arise and pursues these through the preceding series of more specific questions. The tone is slightly more confrontational and at times humorous but remains for the most part one that aims to make the family comfortable with this process. Because this is a brief phase of therapy in which most problems of adolescence cannot be resolved, it is important for the therapist not to raise such an expectation in the family; instead, the family should feel encouraged that they will be able to manage such problems or issues if they arise.

THERAPIST: One of the things that anorexia does—the reason I'm focusing on this so much—is change how someone might approach things as an adolescent. I think the strategies you (*to the parents*) are describing to manage these kinds of issues in adolescence are excellent. But anorexia, as you noted, can put all those things off track. Suddenly her body wasn't working like an adolescent body anymore, it was working like a preadolescent body. You know, she got thin, she didn't look like an adolescent, she stopped having her menses, her social life completely declined, she became withdrawn, so she wasn't working on those issues and developing that part of her that is essential to becoming an adult. And her interest in boys was undeveloped. Bobby comes over, it's new, so that part of herself in sexual development and part of herself that is interested in love and romance is also sort of lost. As were career aspirations also, but a little bit less.

RHONDA: Well, I noticed, when I just started declining my meals, I got very short, short patience, I was on edge a lot. And sometimes I would be like that with my friends, and I didn't mean to, I just was.

MOTHER: It was your parents, too.

RHONDA: Parents, too, but it was more so, I don't know, it was like, I didn't want to, I guess, put up with anything. Because I was, I don't know, I guess I just wasn't getting energy to my brain, so I was. . . .

MOTHER: Also in class, you said you would think about calories you were going to eat during that day.

RHONDA: Right, and I wouldn't concentrate on my schoolwork

MOTHER: Then your mind would wander.

THERAPIST: So you can see how important it is in part of recovery from the illness to make sure that those kinds of things get back on track. And it sounds like, from a parental perspective, because you have had to be parents of someone who seemed much younger, much more than you had to be, even last summer. You have really had to come in and help with her health problems and not eating. And now adolescence is back, hopefully it will stay back on all fronts, right?

RHONDA: Also, to say something else, that, also when you stop eating, too, it's kind of like when I talk on the phone or something, I didn't know, "Oh, am I going to talk to this one tonight, or should I call this one?" It wasn't a routine, I never really had a routine. But then once I was, I stopped eating some meals, or I just ate something here and there. I would have a routine, where I go to school, then I go to my horse, and then I come home. And the next day I go to school, horse, home. And I do those routines every day, and

I didn't want to get out of a routine. And it was more or less why I was on edge, because if someone called me unexpectedly, or if someone was talking to me, it was kind of like, how I was thinking, "Why are you trying to disrupt me? Why are you trying to distract me, why are you trying to take me away from thinking about calories?" I didn't plan that. And that was maybe why I was on edge too, because while I was thinking about calories, I didn't want to have someone talking to me, or me thinking about something else.

FATHER: Distract you.

RHONDA: Distract me, so that's maybe why.

THERAPIST: Well, everyone can get out of sync as a result of the illness. You get out of sync in terms of your development, as you pointed out, because of all these things. Your body is not working as well, you're irritable, you're short-tempered, your interest in other people is less, you focus on routines and calories, you as parents get concerned and worried and anxious, and you have to figure out how to deal with that. So it changes a lot. So now we are kind of trying to move it back forward to where it is back working the way it should, and the way you want it to as a family.

In the foregoing interventions, the therapist relates the issues of adolescence to the past eating-disorder symptoms. This could be done in earlier sessions, prior to the formal review, but overall it works as a strategy to begin to "tie the therapy together" as termination approaches.

Checking How Much the Parents Are Doing as a Couple

THERAPIST: One of the things I'd like to ask of this process, and I've asked it a little bit before, I'll ask it again, just as a sort of checking point, is, what have the two of you (*to parents*) done on your own lately? What kind of activity have you two done on your own to stimulate your own relationship?

MOTHER: You mean as far as Rhonda . . . ?

THERAPIST: As a couple.

MOTHER: Oh, as a couple. Nothing out of the ordinary.

THERAPIST: It doesn't have to be special, I'm just saying anything.

MOTHER: We've been walking more.

FATHER: Not as a couple, he's talking as a couple. Oh, no, we do, we do.

MOTHER: A couple times when Rhonda. . . .

FATHER: When Rhonda is riding and she comes home late.

MOTHER: But most of the time, the three of us, I don't know, ever since Rhonda could walk or something, we do stuff together, the three of us.

FATHER: Yeah, when Rhonda is out on her own, we just make our own plans. If we want to go to dinner, we go to dinner, or go visit somebody. I can't pick anything out.

MOTHER: We're not the type of people, you know, like a husband and wife, their kids are grown now, they have families of their own, "Okay, now what do we do?"

FATHER: They fall apart.

MOTHER: They fall apart, see, we wouldn't do that because we're together. If Rhonda is not with us, we do things together. If she's with us, the three of us, we're the Three Musketeers half the time.

FATHER: See, change to me should be good.

THERAPIST: 'Course it can.

FATHER: To me, I'm not a worrywart. If something happens, I'll deal with it, but I'm not going to worry about it. Because you could go 100, 200 years, you'd be worrying about it, you'll kill yourself worrying about it, and it may never take place, but deal with something as it turns up. And if it's change, it's probably for the better, or for good.

THERAPIST: In this case, I'm trying to encourage you to think about this as an opportunity to help set things right again with adolescence. This is why I'm asking these questions. It's not to tell you what to do, or to worry you about things that aren't so. One of the ways that I, one of the things that happens and I think needs to happen . . . it's not that I'm worried about you as a couple, it's that I think I'd like to see that part happening at the same time, more of Rhonda involved in other things. Partly to encourage Rhonda to do other things, too, and partly to allow you to let her do them.

FATHER: You mean thinking that in Rhonda's mind, she feels like she has to be there as part of us? Is that what you're saying?

THERAPIST: Not necessarily.

FATHER: Because I don't think that even enters her mind, really.

MOTHER: If she doesn't want to do anything with us, she won't.

FATHER: Because we've gone through a lot of years of our life single and married. We know how to live and do what we want to do, we've always been very independent, always.

THERAPIST: Well, I would like you to consider just making a special effort to do something, sometime between now and the next time we meet. It's a very special effort for the two of you, not just that it happens accidentally, but that it's conscious. Doesn't exclude doing all the other things that you would normally do, but this is one conscious decision.

MOTHER: To do as a couple, just a couple only, and Rhonda is out of it?

THERAPIST: Yeah, just one time.

MOTHER: I know, we could go to Hawaii, and leave Rhonda (*laughing*).

FATHER: I was just thinking that.

RHONDA: Don't you dare.

FATHER: We'll leave her when we go on vacation.

RHONDA: Don't you dare, I would be mad.

MOTHER: We wouldn't do that, Rhonda.

THERAPIST: That would be dramatic, especially since you already have her ticket.

FATHER: Yeah, we would lose money if she doesn't go, or we'd have to take somebody else, you can't do it anymore, either, with the airlines.

MOTHER: No, you have to show picture ID.

THERAPIST: They're really working it out, they're saying, "Hmm, who could we take that looks like Rhonda?"

RHONDA: My horse, hmm.

THERAPIST: Well, let me end the session, I've got to recommend that to you, it could be while you're in Hawaii.

These exchanges are the therapist's attempts to explore the relative strength of the parental dyad apart from their role as parents. In this case, the parents struggle initially to identify a need for such a role. However, with continued prompting from the therapist, there is a suggestion that they will be able to find such a role, though it may come about slowly. The therapist ends these exchanges with a recommendation to undertake a specific activity together as a couple while they are on vacation with their daughter. Although such directive action is unusual, the therapist wishes to emphasize the importance of exploring their relationship apart from their daughter.

Planning for Future Issues

RHONDA: Actually, they did do things when we went on the cruise in August to Alaska, because I met people.

FATHER: Yeah, we never were with her.

RHONDA: Yeah, I was with them most of the time.

FATHER: She got up late in the morning, we got up and had breakfast.

THERAPIST: Yeah, but that was a little before all this started.

FATHER: No . . . it was in the start.

MOTHER: But we weren't aware of it.

FATHER: Not yet.

THERAPIST: That's what I mean. It probably. . . . Umm, okay, so you're going to Hawaii, you're graduating. How's that?

RHONDA: I have this week, dead week just studying.

THERAPIST: You have to study?

RHONDA: Yeah.

FATHER: That's 2 weeks from today.

MOTHER: June 11.

RHONDA: So we have just 2 more weeks, less than 2 more weeks, because I only have 4 days of this coming week, and then, 4 days of the next week, so 8 days.

THERAPIST: So, your graduation is 2 weeks from today?

RHONDA: Yes, 7:00.

THERAPIST: That's absolutely wonderful, I know there was a shock, because there was a chance that you may not get to graduate, because of the illness and the hospital.

MOTHER: Well, she missed a lot of school, but I kept in very close contact with her counselor, and with one of the vice principals of counseling, Ms. [X]. She would send memos to all the teachers saying, "Please give work for her mother to bring to her." I would coordinate everything, and make sure she would at least keep in line with everything, keep in touch.

THERAPIST: Well, that's terrific that all of you helped her, and Rhonda has been able to do the work. That's wonderful. And next week you are going to Hawaii?

FATHER: It's sort of strange because we couldn't get in from the weekend to another weekend, so we're leaving on a Monday, and coming back the following Tuesday.

MOTHER: Because of the airlines.

FATHER: We won't be back actually until the 29th, the very end of June.

THERAPIST: And, let's see, what are you doing after you get back for the rest of the summer?

RHONDA: Umm, by that time I'm going to be riding.

THERAPIST: That's your goal?

RHONDA: I'm going to be riding the whole time, that's my summer. And be with . . . my only close friend who is going away is Laura. I'll probably bring her up there, because she has never seen me ride, she has never seen the horse.

THERAPIST: So you're not planning to do work? And when does college start?

RHONDA: The 23rd, I think.

The therapist adopts an upbeat and encouraging tone. The aim is to help the family feel confident that the progress that they have seen so far can and will continue as long as they continue to do as they are doing. There will be a long time between this session and the next session, which will be the termination session. Thus the therapist wishes to instill such hope clearly, as well as to communicate his confidence that they will succeed.

Summarizing the Session

There is still an additional session that will be used for termination, so it is not illustrated in this case.

THERAPIST: So let me just summarize the session. First of all, Rhonda is continuing to do very well in her weight. The two of you have backed off completely from managing this, and that is going very well. And your only goal right now is to really get your menses back, get her whole body back into it, her bones, everything. Which is terrific. Second, we talked about general tasks of adolescence, we went over the past before Rhonda was sick, and how it has been affected by the illness, and we went over some of the issues that I wanted just to bring to the fore. And then, third, we talked a little about the future and what it contains. What I would like to recommend is that I see you in 2 months, to me that sounds about right now. You're going to be gone for more or less a month with activities, and I think that things are going well enough that 2 months is adequate, and it's typical of what would happen at this point.

14

Summary of a Completed Case

*T*he case presented here demonstrates how the family's help can be solicited in restoring the adolescent's health in much the same way as if the patient had been admitted to a specialist inpatient facility. Although the treatment in this case was relatively uncomplicated and brief, the family had to overcome their initial exasperation with the patient's self-starvation in order to be helpful in the process of her weight restoration. When this initial stumbling block was resolved, in part by the therapist's modeling of an uncritical stance toward the patient's dilemma, the family was successful in nurturing their daughter back to health. Once her weight was restored and the adolescent reintegrated with her peer group, she could negotiate her continued individuation with her parents, but without the eating disorder to cloud their relationship.

Case Illustration

Presenting Problem/Client Description

Sarah was a 15-year-old 10th-grade adolescent with a 6-month history of food restriction, excessive exercise, and weight loss (25 pounds in 6 months). Prior to beginning therapy, Sarah was evaluated and found

A version of this case was first published by Le Grange (1999). Copyright 1999 by John Wiley & Sons, Inc. Adapted by permission.

to meet diagnostic criteria for AN. Sarah's mother, a health care worker, made the call to the office expressing concern about Sarah's precipitous weight loss and urge to exercise at every opportunity and the fact that she was becoming more withdrawn. Her pediatrician had seen Sarah a few times prior to her mother's call. Routine laboratory investigations showed no abnormalities, but the pediatrician shared the mother's concern about Sarah's weight loss. Her mother had also taken Sarah to a counselor in the past month to discuss Sarah's difficulties, but Sarah experienced the session as an invasion of privacy and decided not to return. The mother said that Sarah's father, a successful business executive, shared her concerns about Sarah and believed that additional treatment options should be taken to address their daughter's eating disorder. Sarah's brother Patrick, 14 years of age, was said to be "very worried" that his sister does not "eat anymore," and appeared "different and isolated." Sarah's maternal grandparents were living a few blocks away, and her relationship with them was described as "very close."

Case Formulation

Sarah's mother was clearly worried about Sarah's weight loss, and although it appeared as if other members of the family shared her concern, this hypothesis needed to be explored. The father's role in the family was uncertain, that is, whether he was aligned with the patient or whether he was distant and left the mother to deal with their daughter's eating difficulties. Although the patient's brother appeared to be distressed, his support for his sister needed to be clarified as to whether he was her peer or whether his role was more that of a parent. Similarly, the grandparents' involvement in the family in general and in Sarah's upbringing in particular was uncertain and needed to be explored further.

Because of Sarah's young age, early onset, and short duration of eating difficulties, the therapist's initial goal was to meet with *all* family members living in the same household in order to make an assessment of the patient and her family. More specifically, the aim in treatment was to make a thorough assessment of Sarah's eating disorder and to focus the family on resolving Sarah's self-starvation, that is, to help the parents take charge of Sarah's eating while getting her brother to support her through this period. The grandparents' constructive involvement or appropriate distance was a secondary goal at this early stage of treatment.

Setting Up Treatment

The therapist's initial task before the first session could commence was to set up the family meeting. By setting up the initial family meeting, the therapist began the process of defining and enhancing parental authority in terms of managing the crisis. The therapist used the initial telephone contacts with the mother to emphasize that there was a crisis in their family, that is, Sarah was starving, the family should respond to this crisis, and all family members who shared a household with Sarah should help in this matter.

Although this may seem like a straightforward arrangement, it requires firmness and tact. Consequently, the therapist began by putting forward a convincing request to the mother that all those living in the same household should attend. The therapist also inquired about the patient's grandparents and the extent to which they were involved in Sarah's care, as she often spent significant time with them. The therapist suggested that it might be appropriate to meet with the grandparents in the near future but that it would be proper for members of the immediate household only to attend the first meeting. In closing, the therapist told the mother that arrangements would be made to weigh Sarah in the office but that she should bring recent physician reports about Sarah's health.

Session 1

All members of the household arrived for the first meeting. They seemed anxious about the meeting as the therapist accompanied them to the office. Sarah was a tall, casually dressed adolescent, coming across as shy, and looking frail, pale and with dark rings under her eyes. Sarah accompanied the therapist back to the weighing room and remained quiet as she was weighed. The therapist's attempts to engage her met with nods and single-word responses. Back in the office, the therapist shook hands with everyone, again making sure that no one was overlooked by asking them their names, what they did for a living, and what their understanding of the purpose for this meeting was. To convey the seriousness of this illness to the family, the therapist greeted them with foreboding and in a style that can be characterized as intense, warm, and empathic. Engaging eating-disordered patients and their families in treatment is often a profound challenge, and the outcome of treatment is affected by the degree to which the therapist succeeds in this task. The style in which the therapist greets the family is complex and is designed to set up a *therapeutic bind*: the therapist is both the deliverer of distressing news and a kind caregiver who communicates this concern in a warm and caring tone.

THERAPIST: Sarah is desperately ill, and you will have to take very drastic action to save her life. You must be very troubled by what's happened to her and worn out by the events of the last 6 months. Not knowing which way to turn to make things better for Sarah must play on your minds all the time.

The therapist attempted here to raise the parents' concern about Sarah as much as possible but at the same time to be warm and positive about the family, thereby reducing any parental guilt. The parents' concern was raised so that they could be mobilized to take charge of Sarah's refeeding. To do this, the therapist made sure to get a detailed idea from each family member, including Sarah, as to how they perceived Sarah's state of ill health. Circular questioning is often helpful in allowing family members to provide their unique insights about family life. Instead of just asking father or mother how much they worry about their daughter not eating, the therapist asks a third party to describe the specific event. In this case, Sarah's brother was asked a question.

THERAPIST: What does your mom do when Sarah struggles to eat, and can you tell me what your dad typically does to encourage Sarah to eat more?

The next step was to reflect the family's comments back to them in such a way that it amplified the seriousness of the problem and their sense of having done all they could to help, without success.

THERAPIST: So what I hear is that all of you, your primary care physician, and a counselor have tried very hard to help Sarah recover from this dreadful illness, and still the anorexia is showing no sign of letting go. In fact, what I hear is that it has overtaken almost every aspect of her life, so much so that she will die unless you succeed in nourishing her back to health.

On a similar theme, the next step was to orchestrate an intense scene concerning Sarah's illness with the aim of raising the parents' concern and sense of responsibility sufficiently so that they could take on the task of getting Sarah to eat. In raising the parents' concern, the intense scene should not scapegoat Sarah as having caused her family this distress or blame the parents for her illness. The focus of the trepidation was Sarah's weight, the physiological and psychological consequences of her starvation, the previous failed attempts at engaging her in treatment, and the fact that the family was the last resort for the patient.

THERAPIST: Sarah is dangerously ill and you have no choice but to step in and rescue her. Most parents have a variety of ways in which they approach everyday dilemmas in their families. You as a couple may have some issues that you differ on, and that is okay. However, when it comes to working out a plan about how to nourish your child back to health, you cannot afford to disagree about what steps are necessary to take. If you disagree about this task, it will be easier for the eating disorder to stay in charge of your daughter's life and ultimately defeat her.

Sarah had had limited treatments prior to this consultation, and the ineffectiveness of past health care professionals' efforts should be treated respectfully but held out as evidence of the dire position the family finds themselves in. To get the parents to refeed their daughter, a task that feels uncomfortable for most parents, the therapist should separate the illness from the patient. In stressing that Sarah had little control over her illness, the therapist tried to enable the parents to take drastic action against the illness rather than against their daughter, who was so frail looking. The therapist therefore modeled support for the patient, who had been overtaken by this illness, while at the same time counteracting or modifying any criticism from the parents or her brother toward Sarah. Information about how devastating the illness is and how hard the parents have to work at combating its effects were clearly upsetting to Sarah. She became even more withdrawn at this time and only lifted her head occasionally to look at the clock on the wall. The therapist tried to demonstrate to her that her dilemma and fear were accepted: her *dilemma* of feeling that she was not understood and that the therapist might be exaggerating the problem and her *fear* that the therapist was rallying the parents to take away the control she thought she had over her eating.

THERAPIST: I am very saddened that this terrible illness has overtaken your life to this degree, that it has taken your freedom away, and that it has left you without much control of what you think and do. Most of your thoughts and behaviors about eating have been overtaken by the anorexia, and the only way forward is for your mom and dad to help you regain the weight you have lost.

The theme here was to show Sarah that although her predicament was understood, the therapist had to remain committed to the primary treatment goal, which was the need for weight gain. To stay committed to this goal while expressing an understanding of the patient's fears is a challenge for most therapists. In showing support and understanding for Sarah's dilemma, the therapist attempted to demonstrate sympathy for her position. However, because it was also important to preempt any criticism of Sarah from either her parents or her brother, the therapist needed to address the family's dilemma of trying to understand why their daughter was behaving in ways they might not understand while addressing the weight loss.

THERAPIST: The symptoms don't belong to your daughter; rather, it is this terrible illness that has overtaken her and is determining almost all of her thoughts and activities. For instance, it is the anorexia that makes her hide food, or dispose of food, gets her to insist on preparing her own food, drives her to exercise at every opportunity she can get, and makes her behave in deceitful ways. In other words, it is the illness that gets your daughter to do all these things that you find so upsetting. The Sarah you all knew before this illness took over is not in charge of her behavior, and it is your job to strengthen the healthy Sarah once more.

The therapeutic goal was summarized at the end of the first session. The reason for this was to leave the family with a sense of responsibility to take on the task of refeeding their daughter, to alert them not to engage in discussions about diet foods, and to emphasize that they should nourish the patient according to her profound state of malnutrition and that Sarah's vegetarianism may have to be suspended until she is healthy again. Sarah's parents seemed somewhat overwhelmed by the therapist's suggestion that *they* ought to restore her health, and it was apparent that these feelings needed to be addressed.

THERAPIST: I realize that you may be troubled, thinking that you have come to me for help with your daughter, and here I put the ball right back into your court. However, we really don't have any alternatives that can secure Sarah's well-being in the long run. Surely we can try and arrange for her to go into the hospital, which may even have the desired effect in the short term. I have to remind you, though, that most patients lose weight once they are discharged, and then you have to face the same dilemma once more. If you can do this job yourselves, then you can give your daughter the best guarantee of recovering fully.

The family was invited to return within the week and was asked to bring an afternoon snack with them, as the therapist was interested in observing some of their family rituals during eating. The therapist's assessment confirmed Sarah's AN, restricting type, weight at 68% of ideal body weight, and primary amenorrhea.

Session 2

The goal of this session was to continue with the family assessment, but this time in the context of observing the family engaging in eating a snack. In principle, this affords the therapist an occasion to evaluate the family's transactional patterns during eating and provides an opportunity to support the parents in their efforts to refeed their daughter. At the same time, the therapist makes sure the patient feels supported by her siblings while the parents increase their efforts at refeeding the adolescent. From a theoretical perspective, the therapist wants to disrupt cross-generational coalitions between the anorexic adolescent and an overprotective parent. The overprotective parent may collude with the patient's symptoms and agree that the quantities of food are too great, whereas the other parent takes a firm stance and compels the patient to eat. The family meal is a varied occasion, as each family displays its own mealtime rituals.

Even though the therapist invited Sarah's family to bring along a light snack, it was evident that the meager helping Mom offered Sarah was inadequate and insufficient to promote weight gain. To get the parents to chose calorie-dense foods, the therapist had to encourage them to delve into their resources concerning appropriate feeding of a growing child without sounding judgmental.

THERAPIST: You have to provide your daughter, who is starving, with the kinds of foods that would restore her weight to normal. Snacks like a granola bar or a plain bagel are appropriate for someone not in need of weight gain. However, to correct Sarah's starvation and help restore her weight, it is bagels with cream cheese, pasta with a cream sauce, or potatoes or rice with gravy that will do the job.

The meal helped reveal the interactional patterns of the family during eating. The therapist did not participate in the meal; instead, the event served as an opportunity to learn more about the family's style of eating by observing their rituals and by asking questions about eating. The reason for this inquiry was to help the therapist understand what potential changes in these activities would be advisable.

It soon became apparent that Sarah was not going to heed her parents' request to eat her snack or drink her juice. For a while, the therapist just sat back and observed what was happening with their efforts to get Sarah to eat. Everyone was quiet while the mother, in a soft voice, tried to cajole Sarah into eating. Sarah, on the other hand, was more vocal and made it quite clear that she was not interested in having what was offered. During their efforts, the mother occasionally looked to the therapist, partly out of desperation and perhaps partly hoping the therapist would step forward and be of more direct help. Instead, the therapist limited his inquiries, asking such things as whether this was typical of their struggle at home or, if it were not representative, to let the therapist know how it was different. At this point, the therapist was interested in seeing how the family would manage refeeding if both Mom and Dad applied more pressure on Sarah. The parents were instructed to make another effort to get Sarah to eat her snack. This time, the therapist showed consistency in coaching the parents by making repetitive suggestions as to how they might act, so as to compel them to gradually increase the monotonous message applied to their daughter attempting to convince her to eat. To help bolster the parents' confidence, it is often helpful to remind them of a time when their daughter was even younger and ill in bed with a bad head cold and they tried to get her to eat or to take her medicine.

The therapist learned that in this case Sarah's mother stepped in to "rescue" her. The father was less involved. Thus the therapist aimed to add support to mother's efforts at refeeding by encouraging the father to join in. As the therapist applies future interventions, he can anticipate this dynamic and use it to make needed changes in the family's approach to refeeding.

THERAPIST: Think back to a time when Sarah may have had a bad cold and you wanted her to take her medicine or have something to eat, and you succeeded. This is because you know how to feed a starving child and you don't need expert nutritional advice. It is the eating disorder that makes you doubt your expertise.

While the parents were being empowered and coached as to how they may proceed at the next mealtime at home, the role assigned to Sarah's brother was one that does not interfere with the parents and their task at hand. Instead, Patrick was reinforced for uncritical support and sympathy for his sister, that is, for establishing a healthy sibling subsystem in aligning the patient with her sibling as opposed to being coopted into a parental alliance that would ultimately sustain the eating disorder. The therapist demonstrated to the patient that her dreadful predicament was understood. At the same time, the therapist turned to Sarah's brother and encouraged him to be supportive of his sister, not in her efforts to be anorexic but by comforting her when she felt overwhelmed by the turn of events.

THERAPIST: While Mom and Dad are working hard to fight your illness and nourish you back to health, you may think that they are being awful to you, and you will need to be able to tell someone just how bad things are for you. (*Turning to brother*) She will need someone like you who can listen to her complaints and comfort her when she feels that things are too rough for her and she gets too scared about eating and gaining weight.

Sessions 3–10

The goals for the remainder of the first phase were to keep the family focused on the eating disorder, to continue to support the parents in their efforts to refeed their daughter, and to mobilize Patrick to support his sister through this process. Unlike the more structured nature of the first two meetings, the remainder of the first phase was less systematically organized, and sessions did not follow a prespecified order. Instead, a combination of these goals applied until the conclusion of Phase I.

The groundwork to enable the parents to take charge of Sarah's eating was prepared in the first two sessions. In general, because of the illness's tenacity, as well as the varying level of parents' skill and ability to unite in refeeding their offspring, the therapist should continue to coach and cajole the parents in their refeeding efforts for the remainder of this phase of treatment. Although the father appeared removed from this process on a day-to-day basis, he was consistently supportive of the mother's more direct efforts throughout treatment. They appeared comfortable with this task differentiation in the process of refeeding, and once the patient learned that her parents were not going to allow her to starve herself, she did not resist their efforts at refeeding. The therapist also wanted to make sure that Sarah's meals with her grandparents were being supervised adequately and invited them along for a session in which the immediate treatment goals were reviewed and their cooperation solicited. They were supportive of the treatment efforts.

Each session started by recording the patient's weight. The weight was carefully noted on a weight chart, which was always shared with the entire family. The therapist explained to the parents how the patient's weight compared with those of her peers and congratulated everyone in the family when progress was made. At this early stage of treatment, the therapist continued to point out just how dangerously underweight Sarah was, even though her weight was progressing well. This was done to keep the parents' focus on the task at hand, because the therapist was concerned that they may take premature comfort from her initial weight gain and relax their vigilance. The therapist had to demonstrate a determination to stay with the eating-disorder symptoms in order to send a powerful message to the parents that, for now, refeeding was the focus of treatment.

THERAPIST: I am really happy to see how Sarah's weight is progressing, which means that you are doing a great job. However, we shouldn't lose sight of the fact that she remains desperately ill, and it is very important for you to remain focused on the task of getting her to eat what you think is appropriate given our goal here.

At most ensuing sessions, the therapist carefully reviewed events surrounding eating during the past week and discussed Sarah's performance on the weight chart. The family's strategies to bring about weight gain dominated discussions. The parents, the patient, and her brother were all asked about events of the past week and how they have gone about the task of refeeding. It was apparent that, initially, the mother would spend a great deal of time explaining to Sarah why she should be eating the food the mother had prepared, whereas the father kept somewhat of a distance when Mom and Sarah got stuck in "anorexic debate," that is, arguing about the value of one food item over another (with Mom usually losing the argument). Patrick said that this arguing would upset him and that he consequently completed his meal quickly so that he could be excused. In the same style of circular questioning outlined previously, the therapist verified each response with every family member in turn as to whether that was the way they would describe events. It was important that discrepancies were carefully examined, as their clarification helped the therapist in selecting and reinforcing those steps the parents had to take to improve their refeeding efforts. Mom's persistence and Dad's support of her efforts were reinforced, whereas getting stuck in "anorexic debate" was discouraged. The therapist should use these initial sessions to carefully bolster the parents in their knowledge of nutritious and high-density meals and to reinforce their efforts to bring about healthy eating and weight gain.

The therapist refrained from setting a specific target weight. Instead, percentile positions were used to guide the patient toward a healthy weight. This weight is essentially a range that the patient can maintain without undue dieting and at which menses is comfortably maintained. Because Sarah had primary amenorrhea, it was not possible to use her menstruation weight as an initial target in this process (for patients with secondary amenorrhea, weight at which menses was maintained before the onset of illness is used as a minimum target weight).

THERAPIST: You have done an excellent job with your two children until Sarah's illness has outsmarted you. Your fine parenting abilities are clearly evident in the way Patrick is thriving and in the way in which Sarah thrived before the illness got the better of her. There is no reason why you shouldn't be back on track with Sarah pretty soon, too.

To reinforce healthy boundaries between the generations and to prevent Patrick from interfering with his parents' task of refeeding, the therapist encouraged Patrick to show consistent support for his sister through this struggle. Aligning the siblings in this way made the parents' immediate task less difficult. Patrick was very worried about his sister and wanted to help at mealtimes, and he had to be reminded that his job was to comfort his sister, while his parents had to get on with the refeeding.

The goal here was to demonstrate to Sarah that the therapist understood her predicament—that she was consumed by her eating disorder, that she felt the therapist had allowed her parents to take away her only sense of identity or power, and that she might feel entirely unsupported while this was going on around her. For this reason, and similar to the stated aim in Session 2, the therapist was consistent in encouraging Patrick to support his sister through this ordeal. In the beginning Patrick expressed his exasperation in not knowing how to approach Sarah and revealed that even though they had had a good premorbid relationship, she did not seem to want to talk to him that much anymore. He was very affectionate during the sessions and often gave her a hug when she gained weight and told her how much he loved her. During the early part of treatment, Sarah was not very responsive toward her brother. Instead, she kept to herself and only occasionally gave him appreciative glances.

Sarah's surrender to her parents' demands to increase food intake, accompanied by steady weight gain, as well as the parents' relief after having taken charge of the eating disorder, signaled the start of Phase II of treatment. However, addressing the eating disorder symptoms while continuing weight gain with minimum tension or criticism remained central in the discussions that followed. In Phase II, though, those issues that the family had to postpone were brought forward for review. In addition to consistent parental management of eating-disorder symptoms, the remaining treatment goals were for the parents to relinquish control over Sarah's eating and to begin discussion about Sarah transferring to another school, as she had wished, and returning to the activities she used to enjoy, such as playing tennis and going out with friends.

Because Sarah's weight gain was still fragile at this early stage of Phase II of treatment, the therapist had to make sure that the parents gradually relaxed their vigilance in the refeeding process. As in the first months of treatment, the therapist insisted that the parents remain relentless until they and the therapist were convinced that Sarah no longer doubted their ability to prevent her from starving herself.

Once Sarah's weight began to approach 90% of ideal body weight, it seemed prudent to guide the family toward relinquishing their control over the patient's eating. After 12 weeks of treatment, Sarah's weight was much improved, and the therapist felt reassured that weight gain would continue even if the parents were to exert less vigilance. There were a variety of ways in which the parents gradually reduced their control over this process. Because of Sarah's age and increasing independence, as well as her commitment to vegetarianism on moral grounds, the parents first allowed Sarah to make some vegetarian choices for mealtimes, while still preparing meals herself. The next step was to have Sarah take care of breakfast and school lunch without supervision, and later on the parents allowed Sarah to eat dinner out with her school friends.

The task of the therapist here was to assist the parents and the adolescent in bringing about a careful and mutually agreed-upon transfer of responsibility in this domain back to the adolescent. Once the eating ceased to be the focus of discussions, the family was engaged in talking about adolescent issues that came to the fore as Sarah was recovering from her eating disorder. The aim was to assist the patient in negotiating adolescence and young adulthood successfully. By this time, Sarah was happily settled into her new school and engaged with her peers. She had also returned to playing tennis regularly, which she said she was enjoying. Also significant was the fact that Sarah had started dating. This aspect of her recovery perturbed the parents, especially the father, in that the boy was older than Sarah and had recently graduated from high school. The parents were keen to protect Sarah, while at the same time cautiously taking delight in the fact that she was exploring adolescence without the interference of the eating disorder. An important shift in the parents' thinking here was their concern about her being ready to start dating as opposed to worrying about her food intake. The parents and therapist could, of course, only fully engage in discussions about the issue of their adolescent offspring engaging in age-appropriate activities because they were reassured that Sarah's eating was healthy and back on track.

The third phase of treatment was brief, and was initiated when Sarah achieved a stable weight, self-starvation had abated, and control over eating had been fully returned to her. The central theme in this phase was the establishment of a healthy adolescent–parent relationship in which the illness no longer constituted the basis of the family's interaction. To establish this entailed working toward increased personal autonomy for Sarah and the therapist's expressed understanding of the parents' concerns while helping them respect appropriate intergenerational family boundaries. Therefore, the goals for the conclusion of treatment were to ensure that the adolescent–parent relationship no longer required the symptoms as an idiom of communication and to review Sarah's plans to spend more time away from home as she was preparing for her eventual departure from her family home. Treatment was terminated after 6 months, when Sarah's weight was at a healthy level and she was on her way to negotiating young adulthood without the constraints of her eating disorder.

Outcome and Prognosis

Sarah's family treatment lasted only 6 months. Phase I consisted of seven weekly sessions. Phase II consisted of five sessions that were spread over about 2 months, and Phase III consisted of two sessions over 2 months. Sarah and her family were contacted for a follow-up assessment about 1 year after we terminated treatment. A student who was not involved in Sarah's treatment conducted the assessment. Sarah's weight had stabilized above 90% of ideal body weight and she had started to menstruate, although cycles were still irregular. She was enjoying school and her friends and was dating regularly. During this assessment, Sarah and her parents were also asked about their experience of the treatment. Both parents and Sarah felt that the treatment was helpful and informative. The parents were revitalized in particular by the fact that the therapist helped them to accept that they should encourage Sarah to eat and that they did not feel threatened or criticized: "Treatment helped us divorce anorexia and the person. This made it easier to cope with and not get angry with Sarah. It helped us to be decisive as a couple and to give us direction." Although caution is always necessary, given Sarah's progress in treatment, her clinical status at follow-up, and the family's continuing healthy management of her individuation, it would be fair to say that Sarah has a good prognosis and will hopefully stage a full recovery in the years ahead.

Clinical Issues and Summary

Engagement in therapy and the family's continued commitment to treatment are crucial for the successful resolution of the eating disorder. One tool that has proved helpful in the measurement of the relationship between family organization and treatment compliance and outcome is the Expressed Emotion (EE) scales (Vaughn & Leff, 1976), which measure parental criticism of the anorexic offspring. In a series of Maudsley studies, it was shown that high levels of EE in mothers predicted early dropout from family therapy but not from individual treatment (Szmukler, Eisler, Russell & Dare, 1985). There is also a connection between EE and response to treatment. Criticism of the patient by either parent at the onset of treatment was highly predictive of poor outcome. More tentatively, patients from critical families fare better in family counseling (in which parents are seen separately from the patient) as opposed to conjoint family therapy (Le Grange et al., 1992). As for Sarah's treatment, the therapist had to be careful to address the mother's signs of exhaustion with refeeding and the tendency for her and the patient's brother to become critical of Sarah's behavior during the early part of treatment. It was therefore imperative for the therapist to model an uncritical stance toward the patient, while at the same time avoiding any blame of the family for Sarah's illness. On cases such as Sarah's, in which parents are critical of the patient at the outset, conjoint family therapy may exacerbate these deleterious qualities of family life and can have a negative impact on treatment outcome.

References

Agras, W. S., & Kraemer, H. C. (1983). The treatment of anorexia nervosa: Do different treatments have different outcomes? *Psychiatric Annals, 13,* 928–935.

American Psychiatric Association. (2000). Practice guideline for the treatment of eating disorders (rev.). *American Journal of Psychiatry, 157*(Suppl.), 1—39.

Attie, I., & Brooks-Gunn, J. (1989). Development of eating problems in adolescent girls: A longitudinal study. *Developmental Psychology, 25,* 70–79.

Baran, S. A., Weftzer, T. E., & Kaye, W. H. (1995). Low discharge weight and outcome in anorexia nervosa. *American Journal of Psychiatry, 152*(7), 1070–1072.

Bliss, E. L., & Branch, C. H. (1960). *Anorexia nervosa: Its psychology and biology.* New York: Hoeber.

Bruch, H. (1973). *Eating disorders: Obesity, anorexia nervosa, and the person within.* New York: Basic Books.

Bruch, H. (1995). *Conversations with anorexics.* New York: Basic Books.

Casper, R. C., Hedeker, D., & McClough, J. F. (1992). Personality dimensions in eating disorders and their relevance for subtyping. *Journal of the Academy of Child and Adolescent Psychiatry, 31*(5), 830–840.

Channon, S., de Silva, P., Helmsley, D., & Perkins, R. (1989). A controlled trial of cognitive-behavioral and behavioral treatment of anorexia nervosa. *Behaviour Research and Therapy, 27*(5), 529–535.

Childress, A., Brewerton, T., Hodge, E., & Jarrell, M. (1993). The Kids Eating Disorder Survey (KEDS): A study of middle school students. *Journal of the American Academy of Child and Adolescent Psychiatry, 32,* 843–850.

Cloninger, C. R. (1986). A unified biosocial theory of personality and its role in the development of anxiety states. *Psychiatric Developments, 3,* 167–226.

Cloninger, C. R. (1987). A systematic method for clinical description and classification of personality variants. *Archives of General Psychiatry, 44*, 573–588.

Cloninger, C. R. (1988). A unified theory of personality and its role in the development of anxiety states: Reply to commentaries. *Psychiatric Developments, 66*, 83–120.

Cooper, Z., & Fairburn, C. (1987). The Eating Disorder Examination: A semi-structured interview for the assessment of the specific psychopathology of eating disorders. *International Journal of Eating Disorders, 6*, 1–8.

Crisp, A. H. (1997). Anorexia nervosa as a flight from growth: Assessment and treatment based on the model. In D. M. Garner & P. E. Garfinkel (Eds.), *Handbook of treatment for eating disorders* (2nd ed., pp. 248–277). New York: Guilford Press.

Crisp, A. H., Norton, K., Gowers, S., Hale, K. C., Boyer, C., Yeldham, D., Levett, G., & Bhat, A. (1991). A controlled study of the effect of therapies aimed at adolescent and family psychopathology in anorexia nervosa. *British Journal of Psychiatry, 159*, 325–333.

Dare, C. (1985). The family therapy of anorexia nervosa. *Journal of Psychiatric Research, 19*, 435–443.

Dare, C., & Eisler, I. (1997). Family therapy for anorexia nervosa. In D. M. Garner & P. E. Garfinkel (Eds.), *Handbook of treatment for eating disorders* (2nd ed., pp. 307–324), New York: Guilford Press.

Dare, C., Eisler, I., Russell, G. F. M., & Szmukler, G. (1990). Family therapy for anorexia nervosa: Implications from the results of a controlled trial of family and individual therapy. *Journal of Marital and Family Therapy, 16*, 39–57.

Dare, C., Le Grange, D., Eisler, I., & Rutherford, J. (1994). Redefining the psychosomatic family: Family process of 26 eating disorder families. *International Journal of Eating Disorders, 16*, 211–226.

Dodge, E. (1995). Family therapy for bulimia nervosa in adolescents: An exploratory study. *Journal of Family Therapy, 17*(1), 59–77.

Eisler, I., Dare, C., Hodes, M., Russell, G., Dodge, E., & Le Grange, D. (in press). Family therapy for adolescent anorexia nervosa: The results of controlled comparison of two family interventions. *Journal of Clinical Psychology and Psychiatry*.

Eisler, I., Dare, C., Russell, G., Szmukler, G., Le Grange, D., & Dodge, E. (1997). A five-year follow-up of a controlled trial of family therapy in severe eating disorders. *Archives of General Psychiatry, 54*, 1025–1030.

Fabian, L., & Thompson, J. K. (1989). Body image and eating disturbances in young females. *International Journal of Eating Disorders, 8*, 63–74.

Fairburn, C. G., Shafran, R., & Cooper, Z. (1999). A cognitive behavioral theory of anorexia nervosa. *Behaviour Research and Therapy, 37*, 1–13.

Fisher, M., Golden, N. H., Katzman, D. K., Kreipe, R. E., Rees, J., Schebendach, J., Sigman, G., Ammerman, S., & Huberman, H. M. (1995). Eating disorders in adolescents: A background paper. *Journal of Adolescent Health, 16*, 420–437.

Garner, D. M. (1993). Pathogenesis of anorexia nervosa. *Lancet, 341*, 1632–1634.

Garfinkel, P. E., & Garner, D. M. (1982). *Anorexia nervosa: A multidimensional perspective*. New York: Brunner/Mazel.

Garfinkel, P. E., & Garner, D. M. (Eds.). (1987). *The role of drug treatment for eating disorders.* New York: Brunner/Mazel.

Gowers, S., Norton, K., Halek, C., & Crisp, A. H. (1994). Outcome of outpatient psychotherapy in a random allocation treatment study of anorexia nervosa. *International Journal of Eating Disorders, 15*(2), 165–177.

Gull, W. W. (1874). Anorexia nervosa (apepsia hysterica, anorexia hysterica). *Transactions of the Clinical Society of London, 7,* 222–228.

Gwirtzman, H. E., Guze, B. H., & Yager, J. (1990). Fluoxetine treatment of anorexia nervosa: An open clinical trial. *Journal of Clinical Psychiatry, 51,* 378–382.

Haley, J. (1973). *Uncommon therapy: The psychiatric techniques of Milton H. Erickson.* New York: Norton.

Hall, A., & Crisp, A. H. (1987). Brief psychotherapy in the treatment of anorexia nervosa: Outcome at one year. *British Journal of Psychiatry, 151,* 185–191.

Harper, G. (1983). Varieties of failure in anorexia nervosa: Protection and parentectomy revisited. *Journal of the American Academy of Child Psychiatry, 22,* 134–139.

Herpertz-Dalmann, B. M., Wewetzer, C., Schulz, E., & Remschmidt, H. (1996). Course and outcome in adolescent anorexia nervosa. *International Journal of Eating Disorders, 19*(4), 335–345.

Herzog, D. B., Dorer, D. J., Keel, P. K., Selwyn, S. E., Ekeblad, E. R., Flores, A. T., Greenwood, D. N., Burwell, R. A., & Keller, M. B. (1999). Recovery and relapse in anorexia and bulimia nervosa: A 7.5-year follow-up study. *Journal of the American Academy of Child and Adolescent Psychiatry, 38*(7), 829–837.

Herzog, D. B., Field, A. E., Keller, M. B., West, J. C., Robbins, W. M., Staley, B. A., & Colditz, G. A. (1996). Subtyping eating disorders: Is it justified? *Journal of the American Academy of Child and Adolescent Psychiatry, 35,* 928–936.

Herzog, D. B., Keller, M. B., & Lavori, P. W. (1992). The prevalence of personality disorders in 210 women with eating disorders. *Journal of Clinical Psychiatry, 53,* 147.

Herzog, D. B., Keller, M. B., Sacks, N. R., Yeh, C. J., & Lavori, P. W. (1992). Psychiatric comorbidity in treatment seeking anorectics and bulimics. *Journal of the American Academy of Child and Adolescent Psychiatry, 31,* 810–818.

Hill, A. J., Weaver, C., & Blundell, J. E. (1990). Dieting concerns of 10-year-old girls and their mothers. *British Journal of Clinical Psychology, 29,* 346–348.

Howard, W., Evans, K., Quintero-Howard, C., Bowers, W., & Andersen, A. (1999). Predictors of success or failure of transition to day hospital treatment for inpatients with anorexia nervosa. *American Journal of Psychiatry, 156,* 1697–1702.

Hsu, L. K. G. (1990). *Eating disorders.* New York: Guilford Press.

Jenkins, M. E. (1987). An outcome study of anorexia nervosa in an adolescent unit. *Journal of Adolescence, 10*(1), 71–81.

Kennedy, S. H., & Garfinkel, P. E. (1989). Patients admitted to hospital with anorexia nervosa and bulimia nervosa: Psychotherapy, weight gain, and attitudes toward treatment. *International Journal of Eating Disorders, 8*(2), 181–190.

Kreipe, R. E. (1989). Short stature in females with anorexia nervosa. *Pediatric Resident, 25,* 7A.

Kreipe, R. E., & Uphoff, M. (1992). Treatment and outcome of adolescents with anorexia nervosa. *Adolescent Medicine: State of the Arts Review, 3,* 519–540.

Larson, B. J. (1991). Relationship of family communication patterns to eating disorder inventory scores in adolescent girls. *Journal of American Dietetic Association, 91,* 1065–1067.

Lasegue, E. C. (1983). De l'anorexie hysterique. *Archives Generales De Medecine, 21,* 384–403. (Reprinted in *Evolution of psychosomatic concepts, anorexia nervosa: A paradigm,* by R. M. Kaufman & M. Heiman, Eds., 1964, New York: International University Press.

Lask, B., & Bryant-Waugh, R. (1992). Early-onset anorexia nervosa and related eating disorders. *Journal of Child Psychology and Psychiatry and Allied Disciplines, 33,* 281–300.

Le Grange, D. (1999). Family therapy for adolescent anorexia nervosa. *Journal of Clinical Psychology In Session, 55,* 727–739.

Le Grange, D. (1993). Family therapy outcome in adolescent anorexia nervosa. *South African Journal of Psychology, 23*(4), 174–179.

Le Grange, D., Eisler, I., Dare, C., & Hodes, M. (1992). Family criticism and self-starvation: A study of Expressed Emotion. *Journal of Family Therapy, 14,* 177–192.

Le Grange, D., Eisler, I., Dare, C., & Russell, G. F. M. (1992). Evaluation of family treatments in adolescent anorexia nervosa: A pilot study. *International Journal of Eating Disorders, 12*(4), 347–357.

Leon, G. R., Fulkerson, J. A., Perry, C. L., & Cudeck, R. (1992). Personality and behavioral vulnerabilities associated with risk status for eating disorders in adolescent girls. *Journal of Abnormal Psychology, 102*(3), 438–444.

Liebman, R., Minuchin, S., & Baker, L. (1974). An integrated treatment program of anorexia nervosa. *American Journal of Psychiatry, 131,* 432–436.

Liebman, R., Sargent, J., & Silver, M. (1983). A family systems approach to the treatment of anorexia nervosa. *Journal of the American Academy of Child Psychiatry, 22,* 128–133.

Lucas, A. R., Beard, C. M., O'Fallon, W. M., & Kurland, L. T. (1991). 50-year trends in the incidence of anorexia nervosa in Rochester, Minnesota: A population-based study. *American Journal of Psychiatry, 148,* 917–922.

Madanes, C. (1981). *Strategic family therapy.* San Francisco: Jossey-Bass.

Maloney, M. J., McGuire, J., & Daniels, S. R. (1988). Reliability testing of a children's version of the Eating Attitude Test. *Journal of the American Academy of Child and Adolescent Psychiatry, 27,* 541–543.

Minuchin, S., Baker, L., Rosman, B. L., Liebman, R., Milman, L., & Todd, T. C. (1975). A conceptual model of psychosomatic illness in children. *Archives of General Psychiatry, 32,* 1031–1038.

Morgan, H. G., & Russell, G. F. M. (1975). Value of family background and clinical features as predictors of long-term outcome in anorexia nervosa; A four year follow-up study of 41 patients. *Psychological Medicine, 5,* 355–371.

Palmer, R., Oppenheimer, R., Dignon, A., Chalnor, D., & Howells, K. (1990). Childhood sexual experiences with adults reported by women with eating disorders: An extended series. *British Journal of Psychiatry, 156,* 699–703.

Pumariega, A. (1986). Acculturation and eating attitudes in adolescent girls: A comparative and correlational study. *Journal of the American Academy of Child and Adolescent Psychiatry, 25*(2), 276–279.

Radke-Sharpe, N., Whitney-Saltiel, D., & Rodin, J. (1990). Fat distribution as a risk factor for weight and eating concerns. *International Journal of Eating Disorders, 9*(1), 27–36.

Rastam, M. (1992). Anorexia nervosa in 51 Swedish adolescents: Premorbid problems and comorbidity. *Journal of the American Academy of Child and Adolescent Psychiatry, 31,* 819–828.

Ratnasuriya, R. H., Eisler, I., & Szmukler, G. I. (1991). Anorexia nervosa: Outcome and prognostic factors after 20 years. *British Journal of Psychiatry, 158,* 495–502.

Robin, A. L., Siegel, P. T., Koepke, T., Moye, A. W., & Tice, S. (1994). Family therapy versus individual therapy for adolescent females with anorexia nervosa. *Journal of Developmental and Behavioral Pediatrics, 15*(2), 111–116.

Robin, A. L., Seigel, P. T., Moye, A. W., Gilroy, M., Dennis, A. B., & Sikand, A. (1999). A controlled comparison of family versus individual therapy for adolescents with anorexia nervosa. *Journal of the American Academy of Child and Adolescent Psychiatry, 38*(12), 1428–1489.

Rorty, M., Yager, J., & Rossotto, E. (1994). Childhood sexual, physical, and psychological abuse in bulimia nervosa. *American Journal of Psychiatry, 151,* 1122–1126.

Rosman, B. L., Minuchin, S., & Liebman, R. (1975). Family lunch session: An introduction to family therapy for anorexia nervosa. *American Journal of Orthopsychiatry, 45,* 846–853.

Russell, G. F. M. (1992). Anorexia nervosa of early onset and its impact on puberty. In P. F. Cooper & A. Stein (Eds.), *Monographs in clinical pediatrics: Vol. 5. Feeding problems and eating disorders in children and adolescents* (pp. 85–113). London, England: Harwood Academic.

Russell, G. F. M., Szmukler, G. I., Dare, C., & Eisler, I. (1987). An evaluation of family therapy in anorexia nervosa and bulimia nervosa. *Archives of General Psychiatry, 44,* 1047–1056.

Rutherford, J., McGuffin, P., Kutz, R. J., & Murray, R. M. (1993). Genetic influences on eating attitudes in a normal female twin population. *Psychological Medicine, 23,* 425–436.

Selvini Palazzoli, M. (1974). *Self-starvation: From the intrapsychic to the transpersonal approach.* London: Chaucer.

Sharpe, T., Ryst, E., Hinshaw, S., & Steiner, H. (1998). Reports of stress: A comparison between eating disorders and normal adolescents. *Child Psychiatry and Child Development, 28,* 117–132.

Shore, R. A., & Porter, J. E. (1990). Normative and reliability data for 11 to 18 year olds in the Eating Disorder Inventory. *International Journal of Eating Disorders, 9,* 201–207.

Slade, P. O., Dewey, M. E., Kiemle, G., & Newton, T. (1990). Update on SCANS: A screening instrument for identifying individuals at risk of developing an eating disorder. *International Journal of Eating Disorders, 9,* 583–584.

Smith, C., Nasserbakht, A., Feldman, S., & Steiner, H. (1993). Psychological characteristics and DSM-III-R diagnoses at six-year follow-up of adolescent anorexia nervosa. *Journal of the American Academy of Child and Adolescent Psychiatry, 32*(6), 1237–1245.

Society for Adolescent Medicine. (1995). Eating disorders in adolescents: A position paper of the Society for Adolescent Medicine. *Journal of Adolescent Health, 16,* 476–480.

Steiger, H., Leung, F., & Houle, L. (1992). Relationships among borderline features, body dissatisfactions and bulimic symptoms in nonclinical families. *Addictive Behaviors, 17*(4), 397–406.

Steiner, H., & Lock, J. (1998). Eating disorders in children and adolescents: A review of the past ten years. *Journal of the American Academy of Child and Adolescent Psychiatry, 37,* 352–359.

Steiner, H., Mazer, C., & Litt, I. (1990). Compliance and outcome in anorexia nervosa. *Western Journal of Medicine, 153,* 133–139.

Steiner, H., Sanders, M., & Ryst, E. (1995). Precursors and risk factors of juvenile eating disorders. In H. D. Steinhausen (Ed.), *Eating disorders in adolescence: Anorexia and bulimia nervosa* (pp. 95–125). Berlin: de Gruyter.

Steiner, H., Smith, C., Rosenkrantz, R., & Litt, I. F. (1991). The early care and feeding of anorexics. *Child Psychiatry and Human Development, 21*(3), 163–167.

Steinhausen, H. C. (Ed.). (1995). *Eating disorders in adolescence.* New York: de Gruyter.

Steinhausen, H. C., Rauss-Mason, C., & Seidel, R. (1991). Follow-up studies of anorexia nervosa: A review of four decades of outcome research. *Psychological Medicine, 21,* 447–454.

Steinhausen, H. C., Rauss-Mason, C., & Seidel, R. (1993). Short-term and intermediate term outcome in adolescent eating disorders. *Acta Psychiatrica Scandinavica, 88,* 169–173.

Stice, E., Agras, S., & Hammer, L. (1999). Risk factors for the emergence of childhood eating disturbances: A five-year prospective study. *International Journal of Eating Disorders, 25,* 375–387.

Stierlin, H., & Weber, G. (1989). *Unlocking the family door.* New York: Brunner/Mazel.

Strober, M. (1990). Family-genetic studies of eating disorders. *Journal of Clinical Psychiatry, 52*(10), 9–12.

Strober, M. (1991). Disorders of the self in anorexia nervosa: An organismic-developmental paradigm. In C. Johnson (Ed.), *Psychodynamic treatment of anorexia nervosa and bulimia* (pp. 354–373). New York: Guilford Press.

Szmukler, G., Eisler, I., Russell, G., & Dare, C. (1985). Anorexia nervosa: Parental "expressed emotion" and dropping out of treatment. *British Journal of Psychiatry, 147,* 265–271.

Treasure, L., Todd, G., Brolly, M., Tiller, J., Nehmed, A., & Denman, F. (1995). A pilot study of a randomized trial of cognitive analytical therapy vs educational behavioral therapy for adult anorexia nervosa. *Behavior Research and Therapy, 33*(4), 363–367.

vander-ham, T., van Strien, D. C., & van England, H. (1994). A four-year prospective follow-up of 49 eating disorder adolescents: Differences in course of illness. *Acta Psychiatrica Scandinavica, 90*(3), 229–235.

Vaughn, C., & Leff, J. (1976). The influence of family and social factors on the course of psychiatric illness: A comparison of schizophrenic and depressed neurotic patients. *British Journal of Psychiatry, 129,* 125–137.

Walford, G., & McCune, W. (1991). Long-term outcome in early-onset anorexia nervosa. *British Journal of Psychiatry, 159,* 383–389.

Wynne, L. C. (1980). Paradoxical interventions: Leverage for therapeutic change in individual and family systems. In M. Strauss, T. Bowers, S. Downey, S. Fleck, & I. Levin (Eds.), *The psychotherapy of schizophrenia* (pp. 191–202). New York: Plenum Press.

Yager, J., Andersen, A., Devlin, M., Mitchell, J., Powers, P., & Yates, A. (1993). American Psychiatric Association practice guidelines for eating disorders. *American Journal of Psychiatry, 150,* 207–228.

Yates, A. (1990). Current perspectives on the eating disorders: II. Treatment, outcome, and research directions. *Journal of the American Academy of Child and Adolescent Psychiatry, 29,* 1–9.

Index

("t" indicates a table; "f" indicates a figure)